THE **wellness collection**

healing foods

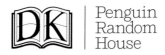

DK | Penguin Random House

Editors Susannah Steel,
Shashwati Tia Sarkar, Libby Brown
Designers Alison Gardner, Tessa Bindloss
Jacket Designer Vanessa Hamilton
Producer, Pre-Production Rob Dunn
Senior Production Controller Isobel Reid
Special Sales Creative Project Manager
Alison Donovan

Content previously published in
Neal's Yard Healing Foods (2013)
by Dorling Kindersley Limited
80 Strand, London, WC2R 0RL

2 4 6 8 10 9 7 5 3 1
001 – 309666 – Dec/2017
Copyright © 2013, 2017
Dorling Kindersley Limited
A Penguin Random House Company

A CIP catalogue record for this book is available
from the British Library.

ISBN 978-0-2413-3412-6
Printed and bound in China

A WORLD OF IDEAS
SEE ALL THERE IS TO KNOW
www.dk.com

DISCLAIMER: See page 48

CONTENTS

"LET FOOD BE THY MEDICINE
AND MEDICINE BE THY FOOD"

HIPPOCRATES

THE FOOD WE EAT HAS AN OVERREACHING
EFFECT ON OUR HEALTH AND **WELL-BEING**,
WHETHER WE ARE CONSCIOUS OF IT OR NOT.
BECOMING MORE AWARE OF YOUR DIET AND THE
HEALING PROPERTIES OF FOOD WILL HELP YOU
TO MAKE NECESSARY ADJUSTMENTS TO MEET
THE NEEDS OF **YOUR BODY** – AND IT WILL DO AN
ENORMOUS AMOUNT TO MAINTAIN AND
IMPROVE YOUR **HEALTH**.

THE PROTECTIVE POWER OF FOOD

Nutritional science has shed much light on the importance of "whole food": we now understand that nutrients in our food work synergistically to promote health – and that processed food, denuded of many of its intrinsic nutrients, can promote disease. We also know of 50 or so essential vitamins, amino acids, minerals, and essential fatty acids that we need to get on a regular basis from our diet, and over 1,200 phytonutrients in fruits, vegetables, beans, grains, and animal products.

A RAINBOW OF PHYTONUTRIENTS

Phytonutrients are the bio-active compounds in plants ("phyto" means plant) that supply their colour and flavour. Although not essential to life in the way that vitamins and minerals are, they support health in a variety of ways.

Antioxidants, for example, protect the body from free radicals, the unstable molecules that are produced through metabolism and exposure to pollution, and which cause disease by damaging vital tissues and organs.

Antioxidants by colour

COLOUR	PHYTONUTRIENT	BENEFITS	FOUND IN
Green			
	Lutein	Protects eyes; boosts immunity; and supports healthy tissues, skin, and blood	Kale, collard greens, cucumber, courgette, peas, avocado, asparagus, green beans
	Chlorophyll	Detoxifying; helps build red blood cells and collagen; boosts energy and well-being	All leafy green vegetables, sprouted grasses, and microalgae
	Indoles	Has anti-cancer properties; supports healthy hormone balance	Brussels sprouts, broccoli, bok choi, cabbage, and turnips
Orange/yellow			
	Carotenes (incl. alpha-, beta-, and delta-carotene)	Source of vitamin A; has anti-cancer and heart-protective properties; protects mucous membranes	Orange and yellow fruits and vegetables (peppers, winter squash, carrots, apricots, mangoes, oranges, grapefruit)
	Xanthophylls (incl. zeaxanthin and astaxanthin)	Source of vitamin A; has anti-cancer properties; protects eyes and brain; strengthens the immune system	Red fish (e.g. salmon), eggs, most orange and yellow fruits and vegetables
Red			
	Lycopene	Protects against heart disease, cancer (especially prostate), and vision loss	Fresh and cooked tomatoes, watermelon, goji berries, papaya, and rosehips
	Anthocyanins	Can help reduce the risk of heart disease, cancer, and neurodegenerative diseases	Cranberries, strawberries, raspberries, cherries, and red cabbage
Blue/purple			
	Anthocyanins	Fights free radicals; has anti-cancer properties; supports healthy ageing	Blueberries, aubergine, grapes, grape juice, raisins, and red wine
	Resveratrol	Has anti-cancer properties; helps balance hormone levels	Grapes, grape juice, red wine, mulberries, and cocoa
White			
	Allyl sulphides	Boosts immunity; has anti-cancer and anti-inflammatory properties	Onions, garlic, scallions, and chives
	Anthoxanthins	Helps lower cholesterol and blood pressure; helps reduce the risk of certain cancers and heart disease	Bananas, cauliflower, mushrooms, onions, parsnips, potatoes, garlic, ginger, and turnips

DIFFERENT DIETARY PATTERNS

While we would not advocate a rigid approach to a particular diet, there are things that can be learnt and adopted from traditional diets. Humans are very adaptable and it is interesting to see the ways in which different cultures have adapted their diets to remain healthy in widely different environments.

TRADITIONAL DIETS

INUIT

The Inuit people of the Arctic have traditionally had very little access to cereals or fresh fruit and vegetables, but the manner in which they hunt and eat their mostly fish- and meat-based diet meets their nutritional needs. For example, vitamins and minerals that are derived from plant sources in other areas of the world are also present in most Inuit diets: vitamins A and D are present in the oils and livers of cold-water fishes and mammals, for instance, while vitamin C is obtained through sources such as caribou liver, kelp, whale skin, and seal offal. Since these foods are typically eaten raw or frozen, the vitamin C they contain – which would be destroyed by cooking – is instead preserved.

MEDITERRANEAN

Another traditional diet that has received publicity in recent years is the Mediterranean diet. This diet is based on mainly fresh vegetables and fruit with some whole grains, healthier oils like olive oil and those from fresh fish, red wine, and smaller quantities of meat. Studies throughout the world have shown that following a strict Mediterranean diet offers substantial protection against heart disease, cancer, and Parkinson's and Alzheimer's diseases. The biggest study into this diet has shown that it can reduce the number of deaths from these diseases; it also found that people who follow this diet show significant improvements in health, and are nine per cent less likely to die young.

JAPANESE

Traditional Japanese cuisine is rich in fat-soluble vitamins from seafood and organ meats and minerals from fish broth, and contains plenty of beneficial lacto-fermented foods such as tempeh and miso. Although portions tend to be relatively small, they are both filling and very nutrient-dense. In fact, Japanese people who follow this traditional diet tend to be some of the healthiest, least obese, and longest-lived people in the world.

ANCESTRAL/PALEOLITHIC

Also referred to as the caveman or hunter-gatherer diet, this modern nutritional plan is based on an ancient diet of wild plants and meat that early humans were likely to have habitually eaten during the Paleolithic era – a period of about 2.5 million years that ended around 10,000 years ago with the development of agriculture. Early humans were foragers who would have grazed opportunistically on seasonally available plants and not made the, often arbitrary, distinctions we do between weeds and crops and medicinal and culinary herbs. Although the hunter-gatherer diet comprises commonly available modern foods – mainly fish, grass-fed, pasture-raised meats, vegetables, fruit, fungi, roots, and nuts – it largely excludes legumes, dairy products, grains, salt, refined sugar, and processed oils, which define the Western diet (overleaf). Studies of the Paleolithic diet in humans have shown improved health and fewer incidences of diseases such as diabetes, cancer, obesity, dementia, and heart disease.

WHAT MANY OF THESE DIETS have in common is that they are plant-based, with meat reserved for feast days and occasional treats. They include plenty of oily fish so are rich in the omega-3 fatty acid DHA. Their overall balance of essential fatty acids is healthier (i.e. higher in omega 3 than 6, unlike modern diets), and they are high in antioxidants. People who follow these diets rely on seasonal fresh food produced without industrial chemicals, which means they eat a wide variety of nutrient-dense foods necessary for optimal heath throughout the year. They tend to eat sensible portions and rarely "snack" between meals.

THE WESTERN DIET

By contrast, the modern Western diet, also called the Western pattern diet, is characterized by high intakes of red meat, sugar and artificial sweeteners, high-fat foods, salt, and refined grains. It also typically contains hydrogenated and trans-fats, high-sugar drinks, and higher intakes of processed meat. This diet, based on studies of western populations, is associated with an elevated incidence of obesity, death from heart disease, cancer (especially colon cancer), and other western pattern diet-related diseases. The high consumption of grains – as breakfast cereals, breads, cakes, biscuits, pasta, and so on – means that grain has become a significant source of carbohydrate-energy, minerals and, in the case of whole grains, of fibre and B vitamins. However, it is now thought that this reliance on cereals may come at a high cost to our health. Modern strains of high-gluten cereals, combined with an over-reliance on wheat-based products and an industrial approach to the processing of grain-based foods, can place a strain on our digestive systems and nutrient balance. For example, an increasing number of people have developed gluten intolerance, or gluten sensitivity, which can vary from coeliac disease to feeling bloated if they eat too many cereal-based foods in a day.

> ## "IT IS NOW THOUGHT THAT RELIANCE ON CEREALS MAY COME AT A HIGH COST TO OUR HEALTH."

Cereals contain what have been termed "anti-nutrients" that may prevent the digestive system absorbing several essential nutrients. The most researched anti-nutrients are the phytates found in the bran or outer hull of most grains, and which is part of a seed's system of preservation – it prevents the seed sprouting until conditions are right. The phytate known as phytic acid can block the absorption of essential minerals such as calcium, magnesium, copper, iron, and especially zinc, in the gut. This may be why a diet high in improperly prepared whole grains may lead to serious mineral deficiencies and bone loss, and why consuming large amounts of unprocessed bran often initially improves bowel regularity, but may lead to irritable bowel syndrome and, in the long term, other adverse effects.

So although cereals can be a useful part of a diet, they do require careful preparation because of their anti-nutrient properties. Many cultures throughout the world have developed ways of preparing types of grain for human consumption. Soaking, sprouting, and souring are very common aids for grain preparation, and ensure the neutralization of phytates, enzyme-inhibitors, and other anti-nutrients with which seeds are naturally endowed. Some traditional preparation methods involve complex, comparatively labour-intensive steps that produce what are now considered unusual foods from common grains, but which were once part of common dietary practices. The traditional sourdough method of preparing rye bread, for example, which was widespread throughout eastern Europe, helps to make rye flour far more digestible.

Modern diets in general also tend to include a larger number of beans and legumes, and, more recently, soya derivatives. Although including beans in your diet can be a useful source of fibre and protein, these foods also contain phytates. The phytate in soybeans, for example, means they are low in calcium and one reason why they are less healthy than you might think, though fermenting helps to make soya a more nutritious food. It is interesting to note that the traditional Japanese diet includes a lot of soya, but it is usually fermented in the form of tempeh or miso. In addition, Japanese preparation techniques eliminate most of the anti-nutrients in other legumes and in grains. Soya milk is not fermented and so can be a cause of digestive problems and calcium depletion, as well as being a fairly potent phytoestrogen – potentially useful for reducing hot flushes in menopausal women, but not so suitable for children or everyone else.

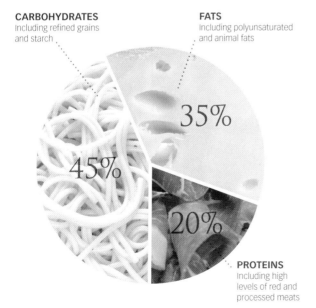

CARBOHYDRATES
Including refined grains and starch

FATS
Including polyunsaturated and animal fats

35%

45%

20%

PROTEINS
Including high levels of red and processed meats

WESTERN DIET FIGURES

In a Western diet, the main nutritional building blocks of fats, carbohydrates, and protein are often processed, nutrient-poor foods high in sugar, refined grains, and saturated fats.

VARIETY IS THE SPICE OF LIFE

The good news is that if you currently eat a modern Western diet, you can easily adapt your eating habits to dramatically improve your health. Including a variety of nutrient-rich, low-energy foods such as vegetables and fruit in your diet both helps with weight control and can have a positive effect on your health: eating a varied diet ensures we get a steady supply of highly bioavailable nutrients that help to reduce the likelihood of conditions such as Alzheimer's disease, dementia, anxiety, depression, arthritis, some types of cancer (including breast and bowel cancer), and heart and circulatory disease.

DIETARY DIVERSITY

No single food or food group can supply all the nutrients we need, which is why a diverse diet is so important. Research consistently shows that dietary diversity protects against the onset of type 2 diabetes, for example, by balancing blood sugar levels and protecting against blood vessel damage. A varied, seasonal diet rich in plant foods can also lower your total risk of cancer and has been shown to protect against some very specific cancers of the digestive tract. To improve the balance and variety of your diet, choose foods like multigrain breads and muesli that have variety "built in", and eat side-dishes and condiments such as fruit and vegetable salads, sprouted pulses, fresh salsas, pickles, and chutneys. Stir fries, casseroles, and soups with many ingredients are another easy way to increase the diversity of your diet. Or when grocery shopping, regularly buy a fruit or vegetable that is not familiar to you to prepare and eat. Following a varied diet also tends to be more satisfying and so reduces your sugar, salt, and saturated fat consumption – all risk factors for heart disease. Including more spices and herbs in your food can also boost its flavour and nutritional density: adding a handful of chopped fresh herbs to lettuce in a salad, for example, can add up to 75 per cent extra antioxidants to the food.

Vary your diet

TYPICAL DIET	DIVERSE DIET	
BREAKFAST Wheat bran cereal with milk, sugar and banana; orange juice; tea with milk	**BREAKFAST** Oat porridge made with milk, sprinkled with dried fruit, sunflower and pumpkin seeds, and seasoned with cinnamon and maple syrup; rosehip and hibiscus tea	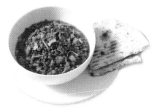 **Lentil soup** p30
LUNCH Wheat bread, ham, cheese, and lettuce sandwich with mayonnaise for spread; a piece of fruit	**LUNCH** Lentil soup *(p30)* made with ginger, turmeric, shallots, garlic and chilli; served with slice of rye bread spread with butter; a piece of fruit	
DINNER Chicken (or other meat) served with a vegetable and rice	**DINNER** Salmon with dill and yogurt dressing *(p21)* served with an adzuki and mung bean salad with tomatoes and a mixed citrus and herb dressing	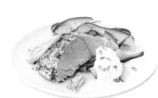 **Salmon with dill** p21
SNACK Potato crisps	**SNACK** Multiseed crackers (e.g. wheat, pumpkin seed, linseed, poppy seed) spread with Hummus made with chickpeas, tahini, coriander, paprika	
TOTAL OF 13 FOODS	**TOTAL OF 35 FOODS**	

As Nature Intended

The success of traditional diets such as the Mediterranean and Inuit diets in sustaining good health and well-being (p5) lies in the fact that they each contain a carefully balanced range of seasonal nutrient-rich foods that are available from local sources. To get the very best from locally grown fresh produce, however, it is worth considering buying organic, as foods that are produced this way contain more of the nutrients that make these seasonal foods so beneficial to our health.

LOCAL AND SEASONAL

Adjusting your diet with the seasons can mean that, as well as being beneficial for your body's "energies", you will eat more fresh foods that can be locally sourced. Choosing local and seasonal should also encourage you to make healthier choices, and can increase a general feeling of well-being as you become more in tune with the cycles of nature. This doesn't mean that you need to become rigid or obsessive about what you eat and when; some foods, such as avocados or bananas, may simply not grow where you live. It is the principles you base your dietary habits on that are key. The 80:20 rule – eating 80 per cent of local, seasonal, unprocessed foods and 20 per cent of more exotic foods, or "treats" – is probably a good guideline. When people switch to more local, seasonal food, many find they become more adventurous in their cooking and eating habits. If you unpack a local box scheme delivery, for example, you may well find an unrecognized fruit or vegetable that you have to discover the best way to prepare, and hopefully you will look forward to preparing and eating it again when it comes back into season. Or you may become interested in learning how to preserve them – a more traditional and low-impact way of extending the natural season of foods throughout the year.

ORGANIC BENEFITS

Organic food is produced using environmentally and animal-friendly farming methods on organic farms. These methods are now legally defined in most countries of the world and any food that is sold as organic must be strictly regulated. Organic farming recognizes the direct connection between our health and how the food we eat is produced. Artificial fertilizers are banned and farmers develop fertile soil by rotating crops and using compost, manure, and clover in order. By contrast, modern intensive agricultural practices have led to the reduction of many minerals and vitamins in the food we eat; official food composition tables in the US and UK have shown that fruits, vegetables, meat, and dairy products all contain fewer minerals than they did in the past. As soils become depleted of minerals such as magnesium and zinc, for example, there is less for plants grown in this soil to draw up, and therefore less for us to absorb. Minerals that are particularly affected by these intensive farming methods are iron, zinc, copper, magnesium, and selenium, and their levels of depletion can be very significant. An early study in the Journal of Applied Nutrition in 1993 reported that organically and conventionally grown apples, potatoes, pears, wheat, and sweetcorn in a suburban area of the USA were analyzed and compared for mineral content. Weight-for-weight, average levels of essential minerals were much higher in the organically grown produce than in the conventionally grown foods. The organic produce was, on average, 63 per cent higher in calcium, 78 per cent higher in chromium, 73 per cent higher in iron, 118 per cent higher in magnesium, 178 per cent higher in molybdenum, 91 per cent higher in phosphorus, 125 per cent higher in potassium, and 60 per cent higher in zinc. More recent studies have confirmed this finding and interestingly, according to population studies, many people in the western world are becoming increasingly deficient in these same minerals, leading to problems such as anaemia, tiredness, sub-fertility, and poor immunity. Organic farming can help to halt this decline in mineral content. Levels of vitamin C, phenolic acids, and antioxidants also tend to be 60–80 per cent higher in organic produce. Just as important from a health point of view is the markedly more benign balance of omega-6 and -3 fatty acids in organic meat and dairy produce as compared to conventionally produced foods.

It is not just what organic food contains, it is what it does not contain that is important. Some synthetic chemicals commonly used in non-organic agriculture are now known to potentially disrupt the nervous, circulatory, endocrine, and reproductive systems of humans. This may be even more of a problem in babies and children,

> "IT IS NOT JUST WHAT ORGANIC FOOD CONTAINS, IT IS ALSO WHAT IT DOES NOT CONTAIN THAT IS IMPORTANT."

whose organs are developing fast. Although most countries now set safety levels for pesticide residues in food, these are based on individual chemicals, and don't take into account the cocktail effect of lots of pesticides, which are known to be more damaging in combination. Many food additives common in processed foods are also banned from organic food products; monosodium glutamate (MSG), Brilliant Blue, aspartame, and tartrazine, for example, are now being linked to health issues and behavioural problems in children. Organic standards also insist that animals are given plenty of space and fresh air to thrive and grow, guaranteeing that they are reared humanely and not routinely fed antibiotics to suppress disease or promote growth.

Organic is kinder to the environment, too. Organic farming works with nature, not against it, and research shows that it's better for birds, butterflies, and other wildlife. Organic farms are havens for wildlife and provide homes for bees, birds, and butterflies. In fact, plant, insect, and bird life is up to 50 per cent greater on organic farms. Biodiversity is something to encourage both in our environment and on our plate.

HOW ABOUT GM FOOD?

Genetically modified (GM) crops provide another potential health hazard. GM foods, which have had their genetic material (DNA) altered to achieve desired changes in their characteristics, have been developed by seed and chemical companies as one means of responding to climate change and a growing global population, although GM technologies have consistently underperformed. There is legitimate concern about how carelessly GM foods have been assessed for safety, and evidence that they may have risks to human health and wildlife. In a recent French study in 2012, rats fed a lifelong diet of a bestselling strain of genetically modified maize developed more and bigger breast tumours, and experienced kidney and liver dysfunction. In the US, GM foods don't have to be labelled, in spite of overwhelming public support for such a requirement in a country where GM-adulterated food is so prevalent. In most countries in Europe, farm animals are fed GM foodstuff, but actual GM foods for human consumption are not yet accepted. Crops that can be grown as GM varieties include soya beans, corn, rice, and tomatoes.

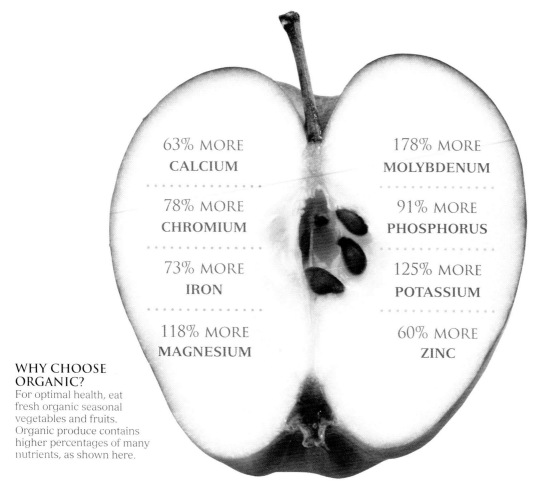

63% MORE
CALCIUM

178% MORE
MOLYBDENUM

78% MORE
CHROMIUM

91% MORE
PHOSPHORUS

73% MORE
IRON

125% MORE
POTASSIUM

118% MORE
MAGNESIUM

60% MORE
ZINC

WHY CHOOSE ORGANIC?
For optimal health, eat fresh organic seasonal vegetables and fruits. Organic produce contains higher percentages of many nutrients, as shown here.

LET FOOD BE YOUR MEDICINE

Food is the bedrock upon which a healthy life is based, and is the body's buffer against the stresses, strains, and the onslaughts of an increasingly toxic environment. Science has consistently shown that food can be used to support long-term heath as well as treat acute conditions. Ginger, for example, is a traditional remedy for nausea, honey can be as effective as conventional medicines at soothing night-time coughs, saffron contains antioxidants that protect against age-related vision loss, garlic helps thin the blood, thus lowering the risk of stroke, and a diet rich in tree nuts can support heart health and even men's fertility. As the cost, and acknowledged side effects, of conventional medical treatments rise exponentially, we owe it to ourselves to eat the most nutritionally dense, best-quality foods. Good food is everybody's right, and in our view the best way to democratize good food is through the widespread use of organic farming and a greater attention to the concepts of local and seasonal. In re-establishing the fundamental link between food and health and exploring the benefits of traditional diets we are not looking backwards, rather we are taking the best of our inherited knowledge about food and farming and applying it to a modern future.

For example, Chinese and Ayurvedic traditions have for thousands of years followed the concept that different foods have specific, healthy properties. Some foods, such as quail eggs, are considered energizing and full of concentrated life force while others, such as barley, are more soothing to the energies of the body. Traditional approaches to food also acknowledge the seasons: of recommending warming foods like oats and spices like cinnamon in winter; cleansing foods such as nettle or dandelion in spring; cooling foods like lettuce and cucumber in summer; and sustaining foods such as pumpkin and carrots in autumn.

The first half of this book will help you to identify foods that have both stood the test of time as healing foods and are shown by modern research as being particularly relevant for helping to improve a health issue. The second half contains recipes, inspired by traditional cultural practices, that benefit various parts of the body or internal systems. We hope that this information will both encourage and help you affirm the connection between food and health and make food choices for yourself and your family that lead to lifelong optimal health.

Food as medicine

NAUSEA

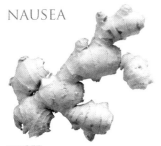

GINGER
has a recognized ability to quell
feelings of nausea.

COUGHS

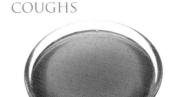

HONEY
is an ancient remedy for soothing
coughs and other throat complaints.

HEART

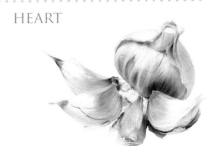

GARLIC
can help your body to fight free radicals
and lower blood pressure.

LIVER

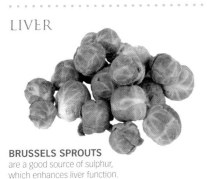

BRUSSELS SPROUTS
are a good source of sulphur,
which enhances liver function.

MEMORY

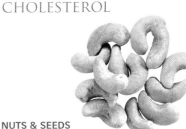

BERRIES
contain antioxidants, which can help to
stave off mental decline.

CHOLESTEROL

NUTS & SEEDS
contain unsaturated
fats, which can lower
cholesterol.

SUPPLEMENTS

A balanced diet is where health begins, but there are times when your diet may not provide all the nutrients you need. A Western diet and lifestyle can also leave us vulnerable to nutritional deficiencies including iron, calcium, magnesium, folic acid, vitamins B6, B12, C, and D. Most governments produce scientifically developed recommended dietary allowances (RDAs) to cover broadly healthy people of any age or gender. These are the basis for the Reference Daily Intake (RDI) values, which regulators use to create Daily Value (DV) packaging labels. RDAs are based on the lowest levels of nutrients required to prevent deficiency diseases such as scurvy and rickets and do not reflect the higher levels required for optimum health. This is why supplement nutrient levels are often much higher than RDA levels.

Who will benefit most from supplements?

Even in healthy people, multivitamins and other supplements may help to prevent vitamin and mineral deficiencies. They also provide more nutrients than diet can alone, so they may help to protect against, or manage, certain diseases. However, the following categories highlight those people who can most benefit from taking daily supplements:

- People who have lost weight, who may be deficient in a wide range of vitamins and minerals.
- Vegetarians, who are more likely to be deficient in vitamin B12, iron, vitamin D, zinc, iodine, riboflavin, calcium, and selenium.
- Vegans, who are even more likely than vegetarians to be low in protein, selenium, and B12.
- People living a typical "student lifestyle" and anyone not eating a balanced diet is likely to benefit from a multivitamin supplement.
- Elderly people living in their own homes, who are often deficient in vitamin D, vitamin A, vitamin E, calcium, and zinc, and occasionally vitamin B1 and vitamin B2.
- Smokers, who are most likely to be deficient in vitamin C and zinc.
- Pre-menopausal women, who have often been found to consume low amounts of calcium, iron, vitamin A, and vitamin C.
- Pregnant women are often advised to take a folic acid supplement, and studies have shown that taking a multivitamin supplement before and during pregnancy leads to a healthier pregnancy and a healthier baby.
- Anyone living in a colder climate who does not get regular sun exposure is likely to be deficient in vitamin D, which can lead to, among other problems, an increased incidence of breast cancer, bowel cancer, depression, osteoporosis, Parkinson's and heart disease.
- Anyone who is under stress is likely to benefit from taking additional B vitamins.
- Many men and women experiencing problems with low fertility are deficient in zinc.

Are supplements safe?

Generally speaking, taking nutritional supplements from reputable companies is extremely safe, but this doesn't mean all supplements are appropriate for everyone. It is worth doing some research to find out about the potential benefits and risks of taking a supplement. There are many sources of information available to help you become well-informed. If you are suffering from a specific disease, it is advisable to talk to a knowledgeable healthcare professional before taking a supplement. If you are pregnant or breastfeeding, only take those supplements specifically recommended for you to take during this time.

While many vitamins, minerals, and herbs are known to safely prevent or treat a variety of diseases, they work by altering your body chemistry – just like any medicine. So before you take a supplement, make sure you know about how it might interact with any medications you may be already taking.

Before you turn to supplements, bear in mind that using the information in this book may help you to replace depleted nutrients by eating more of a certain food. For example, if you need to replace lost potassium, you may choose to eat more bananas or drink coconut water, or eat more fresh berries to increase your vitamin C intake.

A Day Of... Heart Health

Many studies have shown that eating a healthy diet and increasing the amount of exercise you take can radically improve your heart health. These cholesterol-lowering recipes are packed with foods to improve your circulation and lower your blood pressure.

Cholesterol-busting Breakfast

Start your day with a steaming bowl of cooked oats, which are full of heart-healthy folate and potassium. This fibre-rich superfood can help to lower levels of "unhealthy" (LDL) cholesterol and keep arteries clear. For the tastiest porridge, soak the oats in water first, and stir in some freshly grated apple as it cooks.

APPLE
Lowers "unhealthy" (LDL) cholesterol and is a source of vitamin C and heart-healthy antioxidants

PLAIN YOGURT
Yogurt is a natural source of calcium, and regular consumption can help prevent high blood pressure, and therefore, lower the risk of heart attack and stroke

PORRIDGE OATS
Cooking oats breaks down their phytate content, ensuring that you receive all the benefits of their nutrients

Omega-rich Lunch

Oily fish such as sardines are one of the most concentrated sources of the omega-3 fatty acids EPA and DHA, which help lower triglycerides and "unhealthy" (LDL) cholesterol levels.

TO PREPARE THE SARDINES

Mix together 1 tablespoon each of cooked and cooled short-grain rice, toasted pine nuts, and currants, a dash of lemon juice, and 1 teaspoon each of chopped parsley, mint, and dill. Divide between 6 whole, cleaned sardines, packing the stuffing inside each fish. Wrap a vine leaf around each fish to hold it together. Brush with olive oil and grill for 4–5 minutes, turning halfway through. Serve with lemon wedges.

SARDINES
Rich in numerous nutrients, including vitamins B12 and D, that have been found to support cardiovascular health

VINE LEAVES
A staple of heart-healthy Mediterranean cuisine; rich in vitamins and minerals

PINE NUTS
Contain an abundance of vitamins and minerals that help maintain normal metabolic functions

LEMON JUICE
Particularly high in magnesium, important for a healthy heart. Its pectin content and limonoid compounds also reduce cholesterol

PARSLEY
Particularly high in vitamin K for heart and circulatory health

HEART-PROTECTIVE DINNER

Pulses are known to lower the risk of heart attack and stroke, as they help lower "unhealthy" (LDL) cholesterol levels in the blood and balance blood sugar levels. Recent studies have also proven that shiitake mushrooms can help protect against cardiovascular diseases.

SEE BEANS BAKED IN A PUMPKIN POT RECIPE *p37*

RED AND YELLOW PEPPERS
Contain vitamins C, E, and K for heart and circulation health

SHIITAKE MUSHROOMS
Help keep blood vessels clear and prevent oxidative stress

BUTTER/LIMA BEANS
Very good source of cholesterol-lowering fibre

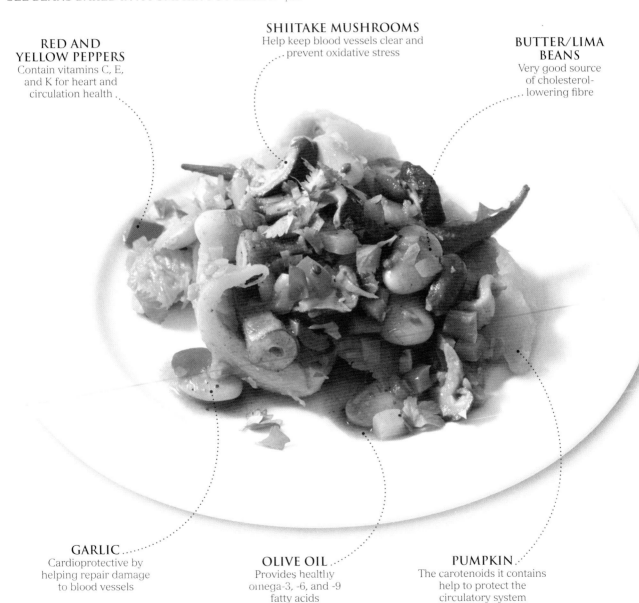

GARLIC
Cardioprotective by helping repair damage to blood vessels

OLIVE OIL
Provides healthy omega-3, -6, and -9 fatty acids

PUMPKIN
The carotenoids it contains help to protect the circulatory system

A Day Of... Good Digestion

In most cultures, good digestion is considered fundamental to general health. Try this plan of eating the right foods at the best time, using ingredients that boost digestive health. To encourage efficient absorption and elimination, don't rush your food, and chew thoroughly.

Balancing Breakfast

Breakfast is a good time to eat a balance of foods: fibre to keep your bowels regular, protein to sustain you, and carbohydrates to give you energy for the day ahead. Top this off with some antioxidant-rich fruit.

BERRIES
A delicious way to boost your vitamin and antioxidant intake

TOASTED FLAKES
Wholegrain wheat flakes provide B vitamins and fibre for roughage. To make, toast wholegrain flakes in an oven at 180°C (350°F/Gas 4) for 20 minutes, turning occasionally.

SUNFLOWER SEEDS
Good source of pantothenic acid, phosphorus, copper, and manganese

PUMPKIN SEEDS
Contain high levels of essential fatty acids and zinc

PLAIN YOGURT
A natural probiotic to keep gut flora healthy

LINSEEDS
Gentle bulk laxative that provides omega-3 and omega-6 fatty acids

Sustaining Lunch

Make lunch your main meal. Chicken provides a low-fat source of protein and assists healthy digestion; here it is rubbed with lime juice, grilled until cooked through, and served with a spicy sauce.

TO MAKE THE SAUCE

Sauté, in olive oil, crushed garlic cloves, a thumb of crushed fresh ginger root, chopped spring onions, and sweet potato, and a spice mix (turmeric, cumin, and coriander) for 10 minutes. Cook until the vegetables are tender. Add 300ml (10fl oz) of stock and some lime juice. Process in a blender.

CHICKEN
Rich in many nutrients including selenium and zinc

LIME JUICE
Excellent source of vitamin C, and can help relieve indigestion

SWEET POTATO
Easily digested source of carotenoids

TURMERIC
Anti-inflammatory that helps prevent gas

CUMIN
Stimulates digestive enzymes

EASILY DIGESTED DINNER

Soup can make an ideal light meal to enjoy in the evening: this carrot soup is easily digested, packed with nutrients, and you can make enough to last for a couple of days. In traditional Chinese medicine, cooked carrots are thought to improve digestion as they contain fibre, thus aiding bowel regularity. The fibre also promotes a feeling of fullness, good if you are trying to cut down on calories.

SEE CARROT AND COCONUT SOUP RECIPE *p31*

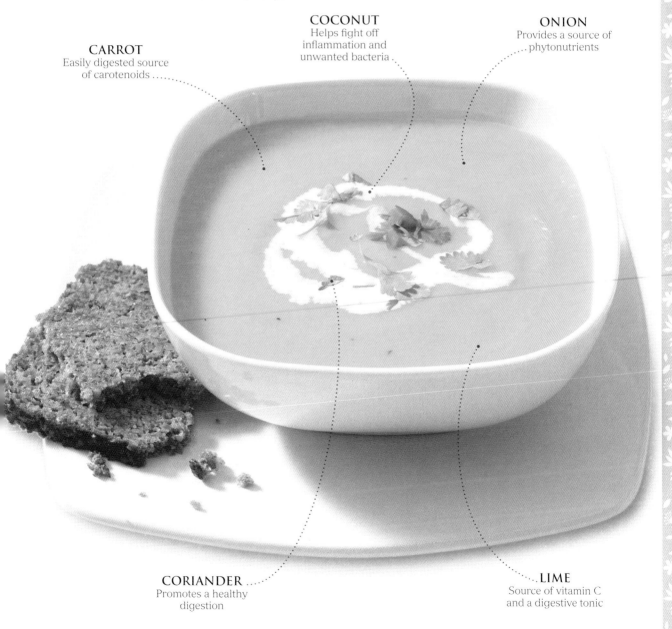

COCONUT
Helps fight off inflammation and unwanted bacteria

ONION
Provides a source of phytonutrients

CARROT
Easily digested source of carotenoids

CORIANDER
Promotes a healthy digestion

LIME
Source of vitamin C and a digestive tonic

A Day Of... Liver Health

The liver needs all the help it can get – it has the job of breaking down and eliminating every dietary and environmental toxin in our bodies. This 1-day plan will give you an idea of which foods can help stimulate the natural detoxifying processes in the liver and encourage regeneration.

Cleansing Breakfast

Grapefruit is an effective liver-cleansing and antioxidant-rich fruit. Combine it with a detoxifying, freshly juiced fruit and vegetable juice for an invigorating start to your day.

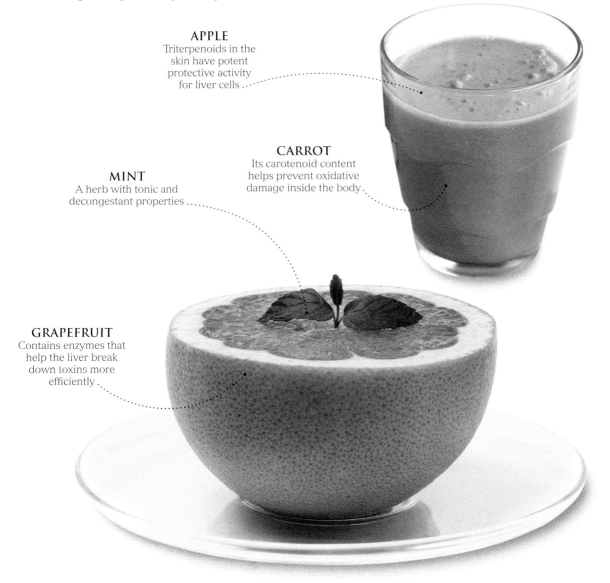

APPLE
Triterpenoids in the skin have potent protective activity for liver cells

CARROT
Its carotenoid content helps prevent oxidative damage inside the body

MINT
A herb with tonic and decongestant properties

GRAPEFRUIT
Contains enzymes that help the liver break down toxins more efficiently

LIVER-BOOSTING LUNCH

Cynarin, an active chemical constituent in globe artichokes, helps improve the proper functioning of both the liver and gall bladder – it causes increased bile flow and is an aid to digestion, making artichokes an ideal food to support the health of the liver.

GLOBE ARTICHOKE
Contains bioactive phytonutrients for liver and gut health

OLIVE OIL
Stimulates activity in the liver, gall bladder, and bile duct

GARLIC
Activates liver enzymes that support detoxification

LEMON
The ultimate liver-cleansing fruit, it is high in vitamin C and bioflavonoids

PARSLEY
A gently stimulating herb that encourages the elimination of toxins; also contains vitamins and minerals

TO MAKE THE HERB ARTICHOKES

Cut off each stalk but leave 2cm (¾in) at the top. Peel the remaining stalk, cutting away the tough exterior. Cut off the top of the cone and scoop out the hairy choke. Squeeze lemon juice into the cavity. Mix 2 chopped garlic cloves, 1 tablespoon of finely chopped mint, and a bunch of finely chopped flat-leaf parsley. Stuff the mix in the cavity. Simmer the artichokes in a pan of water over a medium heat for 30 minutes or until tender. Ensure they stay upright in the pan.

REGENERATIVE DINNER

In traditional Chinese medicine, the liver is strengthened by eating sour-flavoured foods and cleansed by green leafy foods. This dish is bursting with ingredients that help the body eliminate toxic substances, clear blood vessels, and enhance bowel movement and urine output.

SEE MUNG BEAN AND PURPLE SPROUTING BROCCOLI RECIPE *p34*

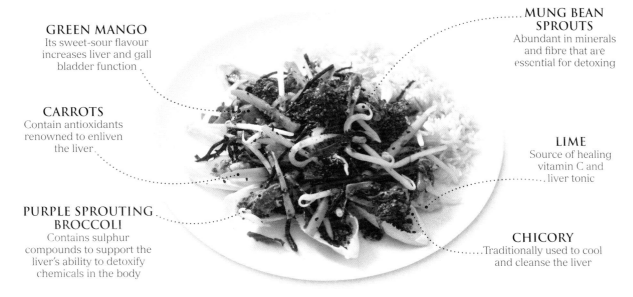

GREEN MANGO
Its sweet-sour flavour increases liver and gall bladder function

CARROTS
Contain antioxidants renowned to enliven the liver

PURPLE SPROUTING BROCCOLI
Contains sulphur compounds to support the liver's ability to detoxify chemicals in the body

MUNG BEAN SPROUTS
Abundant in minerals and fibre that are essential for detoxing

LIME
Source of healing vitamin C and liver tonic

CHICORY
Traditionally used to cool and cleanse the liver

A Day Of... Skin Health

Choosing foods that are packed with the vitamins and minerals your skin needs will, over time, actively nourish your skin and dramatically boost its appearance. Start with this day of delicious meals and build from there, selecting skin-friendly foods and turning them into tasty recipes.

Collagen-boosting Breakfast

Eggs are powerhouses of nutrients that are beneficial for the skin. They include collagen-building protein, vitamin A, omega fatty acids, and carotenoids to protect against UV ageing. Cook scrambled eggs with chopped fresh herbs to add valuable antioxidants.

CHIVES
Contain detoxifying sulphur and anti-inflammatory quercetin

TURMERIC
Excellent antioxidant properties to prevent free-radical damage

EGGS
Choline and lutein help promote skin elasticity and prevent wrinkles

MARJORAM
Popular Mediterranean herb with antiseptic and anti-inflammatory properties

Omega-rich Lunch

Oil-rich cold-water fish, such as salmon, are a real superfood when it comes to skin health: their anti-inflammatory properties help to improve dry skin and relieve eczema and psoriasis. Serving baked salmon in a salad with a yogurt dressing is a great way of getting many of the nutrients your skin needs.

TO MAKE THE SALAD DRESSING

Mix together the juice of 1 orange and ½ tablespoon each of chopped hazelnuts, sherry vinegar, plain yogurt, and hazelnut oil.

PLAIN YOGURT
Contains protein and zinc for skin health

HAZELNUTS
Good source of vitamins and minerals for healthy hair, skin, and nails

SALMON
Contains omega oils to keep skin elastic and prevent wrinkles

LAMB'S LETTUCE
Its antioxidants prevent free-radical damage

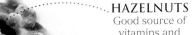

RADIANCE-BOOSTING DINNER

Eating fresh, young green vegetables regularly is a good way to cleanse the body and keep the complexion clear. Include asparagus, as it stimulates the digestion by acting as a prebiotic and contains compounds that have an anti-inflammatory effect and help to prevent the signs of ageing.

SEE STIR-FRIED SPRING VEGETABLES RECIPE *p33*

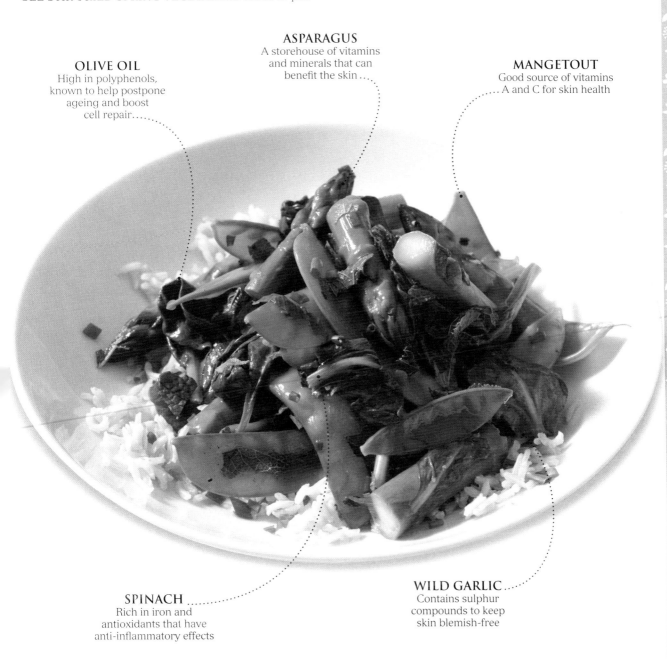

ASPARAGUS
A storehouse of vitamins and minerals that can benefit the skin…

OLIVE OIL
High in polyphenols, known to help postpone ageing and boost cell repair…

MANGETOUT
Good source of vitamins A and C for skin health

SPINACH
Rich in iron and antioxidants that have anti-inflammatory effects

WILD GARLIC
Contains sulphur compounds to keep skin blemish-free

A Day Of... Healthy Joints

To reduce the inflammation and pain associated with arthritis and joint problems, switch to a diet that contains foods known to reduce inflammation and cleansing foods that help remove the toxins which aggravate the problem. Sample this 1-day plan to learn which foods to incorporate into your diet.

Easy-mover Breakfast

Fruit is a source of antioxidants that helps rid the body of cell-damaging free radicals and suppresses inflammation (avoid oranges, as they may make some arthritis pain worse). Apple (fresh or dried) is particularly good for joint problems, but keep its skin on, as this is what contains many of the best nutrients. Serve with buckwheat grains, toasted in a medium oven until golden, and plain yogurt.

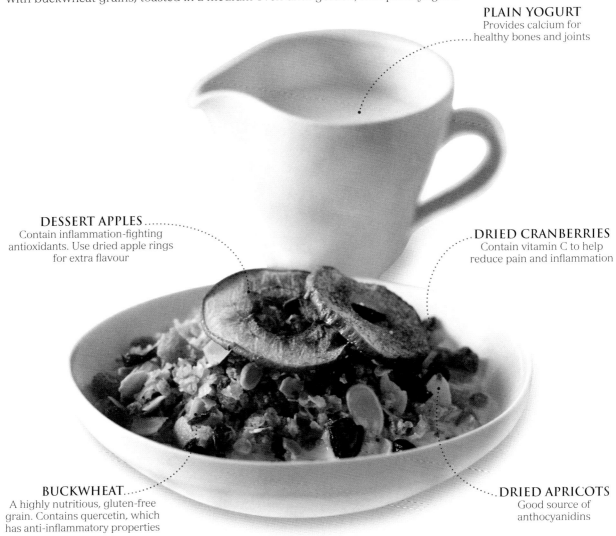

PLAIN YOGURT
Provides calcium for healthy bones and joints

DESSERT APPLES
Contain inflammation-fighting antioxidants. Use dried apple rings for extra flavour

DRIED CRANBERRIES
Contain vitamin C to help reduce pain and inflammation

BUCKWHEAT
A highly nutritious, gluten-free grain. Contains quercetin, which has anti-inflammatory properties

DRIED APRICOTS
Good source of anthocyanidins

JOINT-HEALTH LUNCH

Cold-water salmon, tuna, herring, mackerel, and halibut contain omega-3 fatty acids, which are potently anti-inflammatory. Bake in the oven until cooked through and serve cold with an apple cider vinegar dressing.

TO MAKE THE DRESSING

A yogurt-based cider vinegar dressing is a great accompaniment to baked salmon. Mix together 2 tablespoons each of apple cider vinegar and finely chopped mint, and 4 tablespoons of Greek yogurt. Drizzle over the cold salmon.

LEMON
A source of vitamin C and bioflavonoids, and can help reduce inflammation

DILL
Good source of calcium to help reduce bone loss, and antioxidants

SALMON
High in protein to help build healthy connective tissue, and in anti-inflammatory omega-3 fatty acids

CUCUMBER
May improve inflamed joints since it helps eliminate uric acid and contains vitamin C

APPLE CIDER VINEGAR
Traditionally used to alkalize the body and relieve the pain of arthritis

ANTI-INFLAMMATORY DINNER

This soup is packed with the powerful anti-inflammatory properties of turmeric and so can help relieve swelling and pain including rheumatic and arthritic pain. Use either dried turmeric or fresh turmeric root in your recipes.

SEE PUY LENTIL SOUP WITH FRESH TURMERIC RECIPE *p30*

DRINK

Apple cider vinegar and honey is a traditional remedy for arthritis, as the overall effect of apple cider vinegar and honey is alkalizing. To make, add 2 teaspoons each of honey and unpasteurized apple cider vinegar to a glassful of lukewarm water. Drink 2 or 3 times a day before meals.

PUY LENTILS
Vegetarian source of collagen-building protein

TURMERIC
Contains curcumin, a potent anti-inflammatory

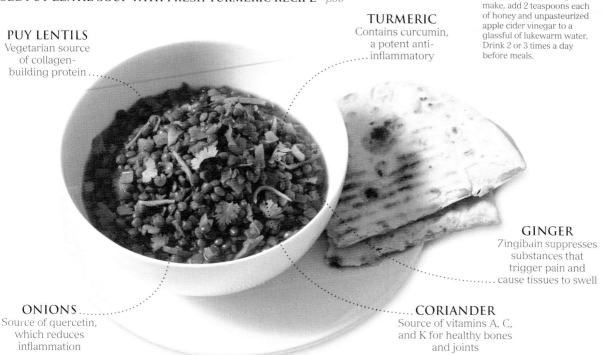

GINGER
Zingibain suppresses substances that trigger pain and cause tissues to swell

ONIONS
Source of quercetin, which reduces inflammation

CORIANDER
Source of vitamins A, C, and K for healthy bones and joints

A DAY OF... BOOSTED ENERGY

Great energy comes from a good balance of rest, exercise, and eating foods that are packed with nutrients to strengthen reserves and provide vitality. This 1-day plan provides an introduction to some of the foods that are known to act as a tonic for the body.

POWER BREAKFAST

Quail's eggs are renowned in China for invigorating and strengthening the body. They are a rich source of protein, iron, potassium, and B vitamins, and taste delicious scrambled with lightly fried chopped tomatoes.

TOMATOES
A superfood containing antioxidants such as lycopene and vitamin C

PARSLEY
Contains energy-promoting iron and vitamins A, C, and K

QUAIL'S EGGS
Packed with 3–4 times the energy-boosting nutrients of a chicken's egg

BLACK PEPPER
Volatile oils stimulate digestion to promote the absorption of all nutrients from food

RYE BREAD
A rich source of magnesium, promoting enzymes involved in the body's use of glucose and insulin secretion

VITALITY LUNCH

Asparagus is packed with energy-promoting nutrients. Stir-fry with other vegetables, such as immune-boosting broccoli and carrots, adding the ones that need the most cooking to the wok first. Combine with protein-rich prawns and cleansing, anti-inflammatory fresh ginger root for an easy yet revitalizing feast.

RED PEPPER
A gently stimulating vegetable full of essential nutrients

PRAWNS
A warming, nourishing food high in protein and carotenoids, such as astaxanthin

CHIVES
A simple way to add stimulating qualities to a dish, chives also promote a healthy appetite

ASPARAGUS
A source of the essential energy nutrients potassium and B vitamins

BROCCOLI
Enhances detoxification, which helps enhance energy

CARROTS
Root vegetables help boost reserves of energy and are a source of beta-carotene

Energy-sustaining Dinner

To support long-term energy, eat a light cooked meal in the evening. Wood pigeon meat is tasty, tender, and nutritious, and is regarded as an excellent kidney and energy tonic. Goji berries are added to give a metabolic boost.

SEE WOOD PIGEON BREASTS WITH GOJI BERRIES RECIPE *p40*

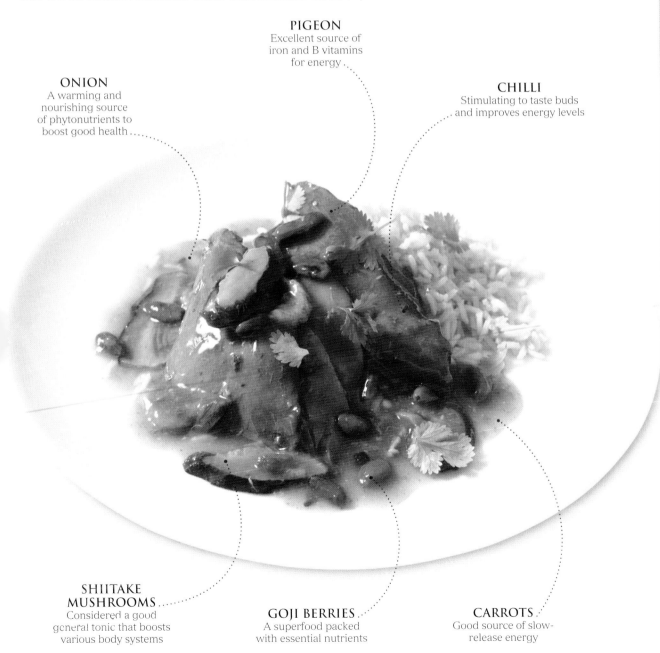

PIGEON
Excellent source of iron and B vitamins for energy

ONION
A warming and nourishing source of phytonutrients to boost good health

CHILLI
Stimulating to taste buds and improves energy levels

SHIITAKE MUSHROOMS
Considered a good general tonic that boosts various body systems

GOJI BERRIES
A superfood packed with essential nutrients

CARROTS
Good source of slow-release energy

A Day Of... Stress Relief

Traditionally, many foods have been known to support the nervous system during times of stress. Today we understand that in fact these foods have an effect on neuro-transmitters in the body, such as the hormone serotonin, which is why they generate a "feel-good" factor.

Positive Breakfast

Eating a healthy breakfast can set the scene for a positive attitude through the day and sustained energy levels. This combination of granola, fresh fruits, and honey provides many nutrients to support the sense of well-being.

TO MAKE THE GRANOLA

Drizzle rolled oats with honey on an oiled baking tray and toast in the oven until golden. Remove and leave to cool. Mix with ingredients such as pine nuts, pumpkin seeds, dried fruits, corn flakes, and bran flakes to taste.

BANANA
Contains potassium to regulate nerve function

ROLLED OATS
A traditional remedy to support a stressed nervous system

PUMPKIN SEEDS
Full of stress-busting magnesium, B vitamins, and serotonin

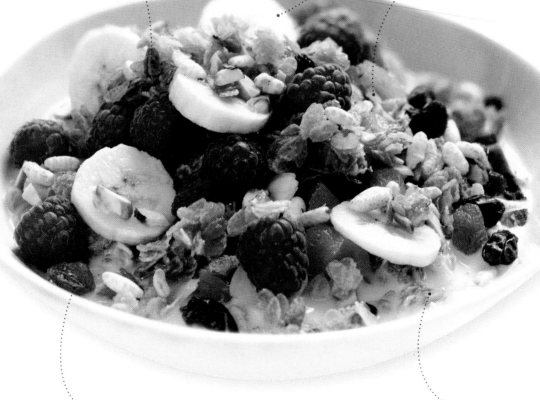

SULTANAS
Good source of energy, vitamins, minerals, and antioxidants

HONEY
A sweet source of antioxidants to protect cells from oxidative damage

Stress-busting Lunch

Sustain your body and mind with foods packed with the nutrients you need to fight stress, such as this fish soup, full of B vitamins, magnesium, and phytonutrient-rich herbs and spices.

TO MAKE THE SOUP

Fry 1 chopped onion in olive oil until soft. Add 1 crushed garlic clove and 1 finely chopped fennel bulb, and cook until the fennel softens. Stir in 1 finely chopped red chilli, a splash of white wine, 400g can of tomatoes, 900ml (1½ pints) of hot fish stock, and a pinch of saffron. Bring to the boil, then reduce to a simmer for 45 minutes. Blend to a smooth soup. Pour into a clean saucepan and add 300ml (10fl oz) of hot water. Simmer gently. Add 200g (7oz) cubes of monkfish and haddock loin and cook over a low heat for 6–10 minutes.

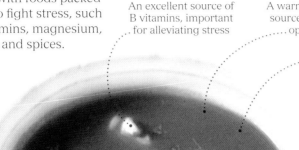

MONKFISH
An excellent source of B vitamins, important for alleviating stress

CHILLI
A warming, stimulating source of nutrients for optimal health

TOMATOES
Source of carotenoids and potassium, for good nerve health

HADDOCK
Rich in magnesium, the anti-stress mineral

FENNEL
Strong antioxidant that contains cell-protective components

SAFFRON
Used in herbal medicine for its anti-depressant properties

Recovery Dinner

Shiitake mushrooms are renowned for being adaptogenic, which means they help the body recover quickly from all kinds of stress. Marinated tofu, which is made from soya beans, is easy to digest.

SEE MARINATED TOFU WITH SHIITAKE AND NOODLES RECIPE *p32*

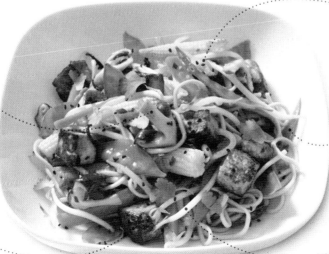

SESAME SEEDS
Rich in beneficial minerals

SHIITAKE MUSHROOMS
Potent phytonutrients increase resistance to stress and fatigue

MANGETOUT
Its B vitamins help produce the hormones necessary to fight stress

TOFU
A good source of tryptophan for stress-relief and better sleep

MUNG BEAN SPROUTS
Contain B vitamins and magnesium to manage stress symptoms

A Day Of... Men's Health

To enhance men's health, choose foods that improve vitality, support the body's energy levels, and are good for the heart and circulation. Men also benefit from a diet that is rich in antioxidants, essential fatty acids, strengthening minerals, and protein. Try this menu for a day of health-boosting benefits.

Fuel-up Breakfast

Start the day with a combination of fresh fruit, seeds, and yogurt – good for your vitamin and mineral intake – or try buckwheat pancakes or oat porridge with fresh fruit. Other suitable options for breakfast are eggs or fish.

PUMPKIN SEEDS
An excellent source of zinc – essential for reproductive system and prostate health

BLUEBERRIES
An immune-boosting superfood packed with antioxidants for cancer-prevention

SUNFLOWER SEEDS
A rich source of omega oils and B vitamins for both heart and brain health

PLAIN YOGURT
Good source of calcium, and enhances gut health

Active-life Lunch

Cold-water oily fish, such as salmon, mackerel, and herring, are rich in omega-3 and other essential fatty acids good for heart and brain health and for keeping joints flexible. Mix cured or pickled herring with cooked root vegetables such as potato (capable of building reserves of energy) and beetroot (particularly good for the heart and circulation).

TO MAKE THE DRESSING

Mix 150ml (5fl oz) of mayonnaise, 1 tablespoon of creamed horseradish, and 1–2 teaspoons of Dijon mustard with lemon juice.

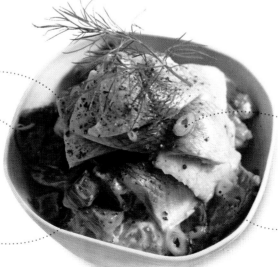

HERRING
A very good source of protein, vitamin B12, selenium for longevity, and EPA and DHA

BEETROOT
Highly nutritious source of magnesium, iron, and betaine for cardiovascular health

POTATOES
Good source of fibre, and rich in vitamins C and B6 and potassium

ONIONS
Phytochemical compounds allium and allyl disulphide have anti-cancer and blood-sugar-regulating properties, while quercetin helps prevent heart disease

HORSERADISH
Naturally antibiotic and anti-catarrhal herb with decongestant properties

PROTEIN-PACKED DINNER

Quinoa provides important protein with essential amino acids and helps build muscle, while tomatoes contain lycopene, which aids healthy circulation. The addition of strength-building walnuts makes this a great meal for active men.

SEE SAVOY CABBAGE PARCELS RECIPE *p39*

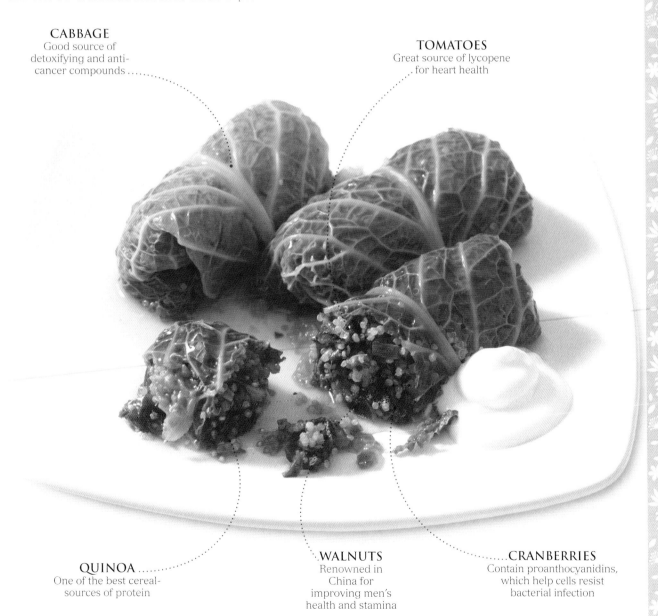

CABBAGE
Good source of detoxifying and anti-cancer compounds

TOMATOES
Great source of lycopene for heart health

QUINOA
One of the best cereal-sources of protein

WALNUTS
Renowned in China for improving men's health and stamina

CRANBERRIES
Contain proanthocyanidins, which help cells resist bacterial infection

A DAY OF... WOMEN'S HEALTH

It's much easier to cope with the demands of modern life if you eat healthy meals that boost your energy levels and sense of well-being. Here are foods that are particularly suitable for women's health, and known for their anti-cancer, anti-stress, nourishing, and balancing benefits.

BALANCING BREAKFAST

Choose a breakfast of ingredients that are full of essential nutrients such as iron, calcium, and the antioxidant vitamin C. Eating plenty of soluble fibre-rich dried fruits, such as prunes and apricots, will also help balance blood sugar levels and prevent constipation.

PLAIN YOGURT
Contains probiotics for gut health and calcium for bones

ORANGE
Excellent source of vitamin C and bioflavonoids to support the circulation

APRICOTS
Rich in fibre, vitamin A, carotenoids, and iron to to promote better digestion, improve eyesight, and build red blood cells

PRUNES
Source of fibre and antioxidant phytonutrients

HORMONE-PROTECTIVE LUNCH

Research has confirmed watercress as a true superfood. It contains an abundance of phytonutrients including substances renowned for their anti-cancer properties, and also iron and vitamin K to help prevent osteoporosis. Try this light yet filling watercress soup.

ONION
Its phytochemical compounds contribute to healthy skin and help prevent infections

WATERCRESS
Contains gluconasturtin with potent cancer-inhibiting properties

PEARS
Low in calories and high in dietary fibre and antioxidants

CRÈME FRAÎCHE
Good source of calcium for bone health

OLIVE OIL
Mediterranean diet staple containing omega-3, -6, and -9 fatty acids

HOW TO MAKE THE SOUP

Fry 1 onion in butter until soft, stirring to prevent burning. Add the stalks of a large bunch of watercress, 3 chopped pears, and 1 litre (1¾ pints) vegetable stock. Season and simmer for 15 minutes. Remove from the heat, add the watercress leaves, and blitz in a blender. Stir in 200ml (7fl oz) crème fraîche and the juice of ½ lemon. Serve garnished with Parmesan.

IMMUNITY-ENHANCING DINNER

Chicken is particularly suitable for women in terms of nourishment and rejuvenation, as it has immune-boosting properties and high B vitamin levels to help the body produce energy. Eat with stress-reducing potatoes and salad.

SEE GINGER CHICKEN RECIPE *p41*

CHICKEN
Low-fat protein and selenium for metabolic and thyroid health

GARLIC
Contains compounds to protect heart and prevent infection

LIME
Excellent source of vitamin C

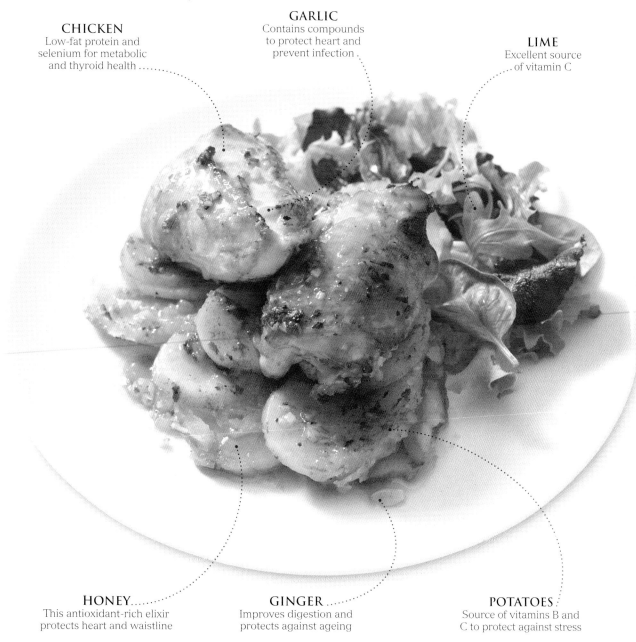

HONEY
This antioxidant-rich elixir protects heart and waistline

GINGER
Improves digestion and protects against ageing

POTATOES
Source of vitamins B and C to protect against stress

PUY LENTIL SOUP WITH FRESH TURMERIC

 HELPS EASE JOINT INFLAMMATION   **HELPS LOWER CHOLESTEROL**   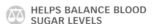 **HELPS BALANCE BLOOD SUGAR LEVELS**   **AIDS HEALTHY DIGESTION**

The ingredients in this soup have anti-inflammatory properties, helping to relieve the swelling and pain associated with rheumatic and arthritic pain. Lentils help to lower "unhealthy" (LDL) cholesterol levels and balance blood sugar levels too, and turmeric helps to improve digestion.

SERVES 4

250g (9oz) puy lentils
2 tbsp sesame oil
4 banana shallots, finely chopped
salt
3cm (1¼in) piece each fresh ginger root and turmeric, peeled and sliced
1 chilli, deseeded and finely diced
2 tsp cumin seeds, crushed
½ tsp coriander seeds, crushed
½ tsp ground turmeric
2 garlic cloves, crushed
750ml (1¼ pints) vegetable stock
4 tbsp chopped coriander leaves

1 Although puy lentils can be cooked without soaking, it's worth doing so for at least 2 hours to make them more easily digestible. Rinse thoroughly afterwards.

2 Heat the sesame oil with 3 tablespoons of water in a large heavy-based saucepan over a medium heat. Add the shallots and a pinch of salt and cook until they have softened. Add the fresh ginger root and fresh turmeric, followed by the chilli, cumin seeds, coriander seeds, ground turmeric, and garlic.

3 Add the lentils and stir until coated in the mix. Cook for 1–2 minutes to absorb the flavours of the spices and shallots, then pour in the stock and bring to the boil. Reduce the heat and let the lentils simmer for about 20 minutes. Sprinkle with the chopped coriander and serve with flat bread on the side.

WATERCRESS AND LINSEED SOUP

 AIDS HEALTHY DIGESTION   **HELPS CLEAR CONGESTION**   **HELPS BUILD RED BLOOD CELLS**   **HELPS IMPROVE NIGHT VISION**

Pungent, bitter-sweet watercress is an excellent digestive and is most beneficial when eaten raw or in soups. It also helps moisten the respiratory tract, making this warming soup is an excellent remedy if you have a sore throat or lung infection. Eaten regularly this soup can help boost iron levels, improve night vision, support healthy kidney function, and improve skin condition.

SERVES 4

1 leek, finely chopped
2 small courgettes, diced
1 garlic clove
salt and freshly ground black pepper
150g (5½oz) watercress
3 level tbsp linseeds and 1 tsp coriander seeds, crushed to a powder in a coffee grinder or blender
2 tbsp extra virgin olive oil
4 tbsp Greek-style yogurt (optional)

1 Place the leek and courgettes in a medium saucepan with enough water to cover the base of the pan. Sweat for 5–10 minutes over a low heat, stirring occasionally, and adding more water if needed to prevent the vegetables sticking to the base of the pan.

2 When the vegetables are tender, add the garlic and salt. Transfer the mixture to a blender or food processor, add 450ml (15fl oz) of hot but not boiling water, and blitz.

3 Add the watercress, 1 tablespoon of the linseed and coriander seed powder, and the extra virgin olive oil, and blitz until smooth. Season to taste, then transfer the soup to 4 serving bowls, add a spoonful of yogurt to each, if using, sprinkle with the remaining seed powder, and serve.

Carrot And Coconut Soup

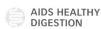 **AIDS HEALTHY DIGESTION**

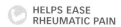 **PROMOTES HEALTHY SKIN AND HAIR**

HELPS EASE RHEUMATIC PAIN

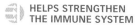 **HELPS STRENGTHEN THE IMMUNE SYSTEM**

With the combined powers of carrot and coconut, this soup enhances the digestive system, soothes inflammation, and protects against premature ageing and degenerative diseases. Carrots are also a traditional remedy for conditions such as acne and rheumatism, while coconuts promote a healthy complexion, glossy hair, and support the health of the immune system.

SERVES 4

1 tbsp coconut oil
3 shallots, chopped
250g (9oz) carrots, chopped
2 garlic cloves, crushed
900ml (1½ pints) coconut water
juice and zest of ½ lime
salt and freshly ground black pepper
4 tsp coconut milk
a small handful of coriander leaves, chopped, to garnish

1 Heat the coconut oil in a saucepan over a medium heat, add the shallots, and cook until translucent. Add 3 tablespoons of water and the carrots and sweat for 2–3 minutes. Add the garlic and cook for 15 more minutes or until the carrots are soft. Add more water if needed.

2 Pour the contents of the saucepan into a blender or food processor, add 450ml (15fl oz) of the coconut water, and blitz. Return the blended soup to the pan and add more coconut water until you achieve a consistency you like. Heat the soup through gently (there is no need to bring it to the boil). Add the lime juice and zest, season with salt and black pepper to taste, and divide between 4 serving bowls. Swirl a teaspoon of coconut milk into each portion and garnish with the chopped coriander leaves.

Beetroot Soup

 HELPS LOWER BLOOD PRESSURE

 PROMOTES A HEALTHY DIGESTIVE TRACT

 BOOSTS IRON STORES TO COMBAT FATIGUE

 HELPS STRENGTHEN THE IMMUNE SYSTEM

Good for balancing blood pressure, this soup also enhances circulation and relieves constipation. Antioxidant-rich beetroot is traditionally used in many parts of Europe as a nourishing food in convalescence, to help combat fatigue, improve digestion and support healthy immunity. Lemon thyme is antibacterial and helps to combat lingering infections.

SERVES 4–6

3 tbsp olive oil
1 medium onion, finely chopped
salt and freshly ground black pepper
1 medium leek, cut in short thin strips
3 medium beetroots, peeled and grated
1 large carrot, grated
2 garlic cloves, crushed
1 litre (1¾ pints) hot vegetable stock
2–3 tsp chopped lemon thyme leaves
2 tbsp plain yogurt

1 Heat the olive oil in a large saucepan over a medium heat, add the onion and a pinch of salt and cook until translucent. Add the leek and allow to soften, then add the other vegetables and garlic and cook for a further 2–3 minutes.

2 Add the stock and simmer for about 20 minutes or until the vegetables are soft. Add the thyme 5 minutes before the end of cooking and season to taste. Divide the soup between 4 serving bowls and swirl a little yogurt into each portion just before serving.

MARINATED TOFU WITH SHIITAKE AND NOODLES

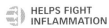 **HELPS FIGHT INFLAMMATION**   **HELPS REMOVE TOXINS FROM THE BODY**   **HELPS LOWER BLOOD PRESSURE**

Soya is a traditional remedy for inflammatory conditions of the lungs and gut. Its phytoestrogens (plant hormones) can also help protect the heart and lower blood pressure. In small amounts, unfermented soya can help neutralize toxins in the body – helpful if you have a hangover – although high, regular consumption can lower the absorption of some minerals in food.

SERVES 6

300g (10oz) organic marinated tofu, cut into bite-sized cubes

4 tbsp sunflower oil

a pinch of salt

approximately 300g (10oz) medium noodles (egg or rice) for 6 people

300g (10oz) fresh shiitake mushrooms, halved or quartered

1 carrot, julienned

250g (9oz) mung bean sprouts, rinsed and drained

250g (9oz) mangetout, cut in half

100g (3½oz) baby corn, halved

1–2 tbsp tamari soy sauce

1 tbsp black sesame seeds

a small handful of coriander leaves, chopped, to garnish

For the marinade

3 garlic cloves, crushed

3cm (1½in) fresh ginger root, grated

1 small chilli, deseeded and finely chopped

3 tbsp mirin sauce

2 tbsp toasted sesame oil

3 tbsp teriyaki sauce

3 small shallots, finely sliced

1 Arrange the tofu in a flat dish. Mix together the marinade ingredients and pour over the tofu cubes, making sure they are thoroughly covered. Cover the dish and leave to marinate overnight in the refrigerator. Turn the cubes over at some point to allow the flavours to infuse completely.

2 Remove the tofu cubes from the marinade and drain for a moment to let the juices drip away. Reserve the marinade.

3 Heat 2 tablespoons of the sunflower oil with 2 tablespoons of water in a wok over a medium heat. Add the tofu cubes and fry until lightly browned on all sides, turning them gently so they don't break. Remove from the wok and transfer to a warm dish.

4 Meanwhile, bring a large saucepan of water to the boil, add a pinch of salt, and cook the noodles according to the packet instructions. Drain the noodles and rinse in cold water to prevent them cooking any more.

5 Scrape off any burned remnants of tofu in the bottom of the wok and add another tablespoon each of sunflower oil and water. Add the shiitake mushrooms and stir-fry for 2–3 minutes, then transfer to a warm dish. Add the carrot, mung bean sprouts, mangetout, baby corn, and tamari soy sauce, and stir-fry briefly. Then transfer to the warm dish of mushrooms.

6 Wipe the wok down again, and heat the last tablespoon of oil. Add the reserved marinade, let it heat through, then add the cooked noodles and stir-fry them briefly too. Return all the vegetables to the wok and mix them into the noodles. Add the tofu and mix it in gently. Sprinkle the black sesame seeds on top, then transfer to 6 warmed noodle bowls. Sprinkle the chopped coriander leaves over each portion and serve.

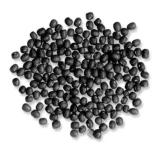

Mung beans *produce the thick, juicy sprouts that are popular in Asian cuisine. They are renowned for their detoxifying properties.*

STIR-FRIED SPRING VEGETABLES

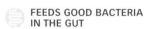 **FEEDS GOOD BACTERIA IN THE GUT**

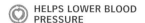 **HELPS FIGHT INFLAMMATION**

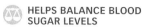 **HELPS LOWER BLOOD PRESSURE**

HELPS BALANCE BLOOD SUGAR LEVELS

Eating plenty of fresh, young, green vegetables in spring is a good way to cleanse the body after the dark days of winter. Asparagus stimulates the digestion by acting as a prebiotic. It also contains compounds that have an anti-inflammatory effect, so it is beneficial if you have high blood pressure and blood sugar imbalance. Young mint and chives gently invigorate the body.

SERVES 4

2 tbsp olive oil

350g (12oz) asparagus, cut into 5cm (2in) pieces

250g (9oz) mangetout, trimmed

150g (5½oz) wild garlic leaves, chopped

200g (7oz) small spinach leaves

1 tbsp raspberry vinegar

2 tbsp chopped mint leaves

2 tbsp finely chopped chives

1 Heat the olive oil and a dash of water in a wok over a high heat. Add the asparagus and mangetout and stir-fry for 3 minutes, then add the wild garlic leaves and spinach and stir until they wilt.

2 Remove the wok from the heat and add the raspberry vinegar, mint, and chives. Combine and serve while hot with steamed rice or quinoa.

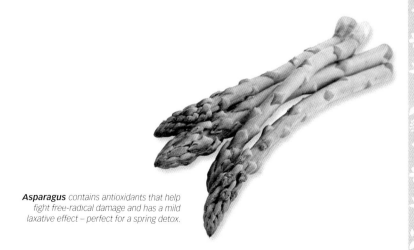

Asparagus *contains antioxidants that help fight free-radical damage and has a mild laxative effect – perfect for a spring detox.*

Mung Bean And Purple Sprouting Broccoli Stir-fry

 SUPPORTS HEALTHY LIVER FUNCTION 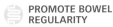 **PROMOTE BOWEL REGULARITY**   **HAS A DIURETIC ACTION**

This dish is bursting with ingredients to strengthen the liver, which helps the body to eliminate toxic substances, clear blood vessels, and enhance bowel movements and urine output. Both chicory and artichokes are known as remedies for issues relating to the liver; in traditional Chinese medicine, sour foods and leafy green foods are thought to help strengthen and cleanse the liver.

SERVES 4

4 tbsp vegetable stock

1 tbsp tamari soy sauce

1 tbsp olive oil

2cm (¾in) piece of fresh ginger root, peeled and julienned

1 small chilli, deseeded and julienned

2 medium carrots, peeled and julienned

400g (14oz) purple sprouting broccoli, trimmed and chopped into florets

250g (9oz) mung bean sprouts

1 small green mango, stone removed, peeled, and julienned

4 large heads of chicory, leaves separated

1 tbsp black sesame seeds

For the dressing

juice and zest of 1 lime

2 tbsp pumpkin oil

1 tsp wholegrain mustard

1 tsp honey

1 To make the dressing, in a jug, combine the lime juice and zest, pumpkin oil, mustard, and honey, and set aside.

2 Place the vegetable stock in a wok and heat gently. Add the tamari soy sauce, olive oil, ginger, and chilli, and stir. Add the carrots and broccoli, stir again, and add the mung bean sprouts and mango, and sauté for 1 more minute.

3 Divide the chicory leaves between 4 serving plates, arranging them in a rosette. Spoon a small amount of stir-fried vegetables into the middle of each rosette. Drizzle with the dressing and sprinkle black sesame seeds on top. Serve with boiled rice.

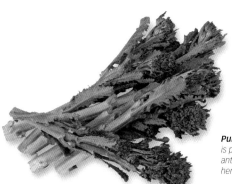

Purple sprouting broccoli
is packed with immune-boosting antioxidants. Stir-frying it lightly, as here, will help retain all its benefits.

MARINATED TUNA STEAKS

 **AIDS HEALTHY
DIGESTION**

**PROTECTS THE HEART
AND BLOOD VESSELS**

Tuna steaks have an astringent quality and are traditionally used in Asia to soothe the digestive tract, while capers enhance this effect. This fish is a healthy choice for the heart if you want a substitute for red meat; its substantial flavour is deepened here by the addition of Japanese tamari soy sauce, which has more complex undertones than Chinese soy sauce.

SERVES 4

3 tbsp olive oil
2 tbsp tamari soy sauce
1 tbsp capers, rinsed
4 tbsp Marsala wine or sweet sherry
1 tbsp wholegrain mustard
2 garlic cloves, crushed
4 thin slices of lemon
4 tuna steaks

1 Place the olive oil, tamari soy sauce, capers, Marsala wine, mustard, garlic, and lemon slices in a ceramic baking dish and mix well. Add the tuna steaks and coat them in the marinade. Cover the dish with a lid or foil and leave in the fridge for 1 hour to marinate.

2 Preheat the oven to 180°C (350°F/Gas 4). Place the covered dish of tuna steaks in the oven and bake for 15–25 minutes. Cook the steaks lightly, turning them over after 10 minutes; thinner steaks will cook more quickly. To test if the fish is cooked, slice through a small section with a sharp knife; the centre of the steak should still be slightly pink. Serve with steamed rice and salad or steamed vegetables.

GRILLED SARDINES WITH TOMATO SALSA

**HELPS IMPROVE
CIRCULATION**

**SUPPLIES OXYGEN
TO CELLS**

**HELPS STRENGTHEN
TENDONS AND BONES**

**HELPS CALM
THE NERVES**

Salty-sweet sardines boost circulation and help build red blood cells.

SERVES 4

6–8 large sprigs of rosemary
8 fresh sardines
1–2 tbsp olive oil
sea salt and freshly ground black pepper
1–2 lemons, cut into quarters, to serve

For the salsa

8 tomatoes, skinned, deseeded and finely diced
1 red chilli, deseeded and finely diced
3 spring onions, finely chopped
2 tbsp chopped basil leaves
1 garlic clove, finely chopped (optional)
2 tbsp raspberry vinegar, or red wine vinegar
4 tbsp olive oil
sea salt and freshly ground black pepper

1 To make the tomato salsa, mix all the ingredients well and season to taste.

2 Preheat the grill to a moderate heat. Arrange the large rosemary sprigs on a grill pan and lay the sardines on top. Drizzle with the olive oil and season with sea salt and black pepper.

3 Grill the sardines for 3–5 minutes on each side or until cooked (they should be opaque, but still firm).

4 Divide the sardines and salsa between 4 serving plates, place 1–2 lemon quarters on each plate, and serve with a green salad and boiled new potatoes.

STUFFED PEPPERS

 HELPS STRENGTHEN THE IMMUNE SYSTEM   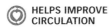 **HELPS IMPROVE CIRCULATION**

This vegetarian recipe is a substantial meal, with satisfying flavours equal to a meat dish. Bell peppers provide a broad range of antioxidant and anti-inflammatory nutrients that help improve circulation and build red blood cells, among other things. With the addition of mushrooms, garlic, and black pepper, this dish also helps enhance your resistance to seasonal infections.

SERVES 6

60g (2oz) pine nuts

100g (3½oz) crimini mushrooms, finely diced

1 yellow courgette, finely diced

1 small aubergine, finely diced

5 shallots, finely diced

3 garlic cloves, minced

1 red chilli (optional, depending on how spicy you want the dish to be)

85g (3oz) brown or white rice, rinsed

2 tbsp quinoa

1 tbsp olive oil

a large sprig of flat-leaf parsley, finely chopped

2 tsp pimentón picante (hot smoked paprika)

salt and freshly ground black pepper

8 peppers of the same colour, or mix of yellow, green, orange, and red peppers

1 tbsp chopped flat-leaf parsley leaves, to garnish

1 Preheat the oven to 190°(375°F/Gas 5). Dry-fry the pine nuts in a frying pan until they are lightly golden. Place the finely diced vegetables in a large mixing bowl and add the pine nuts, rice, quinoa, olive oil, and parsley. Sprinkle in the hot smoked paprika and season, then combine the ingredients well.

2 Using a sharp knife, carefully remove the stalk and the "seeded heart" from each pepper so they remain whole. Stuff each pepper with the vegetable mix, making sure that each pepper is sufficiently filled (the vegetables in the stuffing have a tendency to shrink during cooking).

3 Stand the stuffed peppers in a deep baking dish or casserole dish. Pour enough hot water into the dish to cover the bottom-third of the peppers. Bake in the oven for about 50 minutes. Once the skin on the peppers turns slightly brown on top, cover the dish with a lid or foil. To check whether the filling is cooking, test the rice and quinoa. If it feels or looks dry, pour a splash of water inside each pepper to aid cooking. When the peppers are cooked, garnish with chopped parsley and serve with a side dish of hot mashed sweet potato.

Beans Baked In A Pumpkin Pot

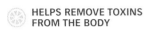 **HELPS REMOVE TOXINS FROM THE BODY**   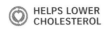 **HELPS LOWER CHOLESTEROL**   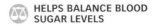 **HELPS BALANCE BLOOD SUGAR LEVELS**

This combination of okra, peppers, mushrooms, and spices works synergistically to support nearly every body system and aids the removal of waste and toxins, while eating legumes, such as butter beans, is a particularly good way to lower cholesterol and help balance blood sugar levels. Presenting the beans in a pumpkin adds extra nutrition, flavour, and a "wow" factor at the table.

SERVES 4

2 tbsp olive oil, plus extra for greasing

8 shallots, finely chopped

1 tsp coriander seeds, coarsely crushed in a pestle and mortar

1 red or green chilli, deseeded and finely chopped

1 red pepper, deseeded and diced

1 yellow pepper, deseeded and diced

3 garlic cloves, finely chopped

1 level tsp pimentón picante (hot smoked paprika)

400g can organic butter beans, drained, or use lima beans

salt and freshly ground black pepper

150g (5½oz) shiitake mushrooms, sliced

100g (3½oz) small whole okra, stem removed

1 bay leaf, fresh or dried

1 large or 2 medium pumpkin or squash (optional)

a small handful of roughly chopped coriander leaves, to garnish

1 Preheat the oven to 180°C (350°F/Gas 4). Gently warm the olive oil in a medium saucepan with a spoonful of water over a low heat. Add the shallots and stir until they turn translucent and golden. Add the coriander seeds and chilli, stir, and add the diced peppers, garlic, and pimentón picante. Add the beans and stir well to coat them in the spices. Season with salt and black pepper and then add the shiitake mushrooms, okra, and bay leaf to the pan.

2 If you don't want to use a pumpkin, simply transfer the bean mix to a shallow ovenproof dish with a lid. Add a dash of water, cover with the lid, and bake in the oven for 45–50 minutes. Remove from the oven, sprinkle with coriander leaves, and serve.

3 If you want to bake and serve the baked beans in a pumpkin "pot", cut the top off the pumpkin and reserve. Remove the soft centre and seeds, and remove a little of the flesh if necessary; the thicker the pumpkin wall, the longer it will take for the dish to cook.

4 Smear the inside of the pumpkin with a little olive oil, season with a little salt, and add the bean mix and a dash of water. The pumpkin itself will add some liquid to the dish. Put on the pumpkin "lid", place on a baking tray and bake in the oven for 1 hour or until the pumpkin is cooked through.

5 Remove the pumpkin lid, lift out the bay leaf, and discard. Sprinkle the top of the baked beans with the fresh coriander, and bring the pumpkin to the table. To serve, dig the serving spoon into the pumpkin flesh so that each portion contains a mixture of both pumpkin flesh and beans.

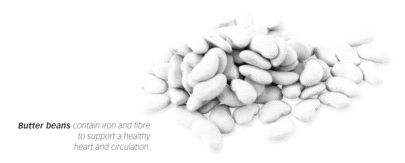

Butter beans contain iron and fibre to support a healthy heart and circulation.

SAUERKRAUT PARCELS

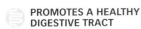 **PROMOTES A HEALTHY DIGESTIVE TRACT**

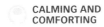 **CALMING AND COMFORTING**

Fermented cabbage, or sauerkraut, is rich in vitamin C and contains a type of lactic acid that aids digestion by clearing harmful bacteria and combating toxins, food stagnation, and wind. Some nutritionists also maintain that it is an effective preventative for cancer and degenerative diseases. Whole sauerkraut leaves can sometimes be found in Polish or Italian delicatessens.

SERVES 4

salt and freshly ground black pepper

2 tbsp wine vinegar

6 black peppercorns

16 whole sauerkraut leaves, or large cabbage leaves, stalks and leaf veins removed

1 tbsp olive oil

2 medium onions, finely diced

3 garlic cloves, crushed

500g (1lb 2oz) minced meat (pork, beef, or a mixture of the two)

125g (4½oz) white or brown rice, rinsed

2 tsp paprika

2 tbsp chopped flat-leaf parsley leaves

300g (10oz) sauerkraut

200g (7oz) smoked rib of pork or smoked bacon, chopped

For the sauce

1 tbsp olive oil

3 tsp plain flour

a pinch of salt

a few black peppercorns

20g (¾oz) tomato purée

1 small chilli, deseeded and finely chopped

115g (4oz) crème fraîche

1 If using fresh cabbage leaves instead of the whole fermented sauerkraut leaves, bring a large saucepan of water to the boil and add a pinch of salt, the wine vinegar, and black peppercorns. Place the leaves into the water, 2 at a time, and blanch for 2–3 minutes: watch them carefully and remove as soon as they begin to wilt. Set aside to dry on kitchen paper.

2 Heat the olive oil in a frying pan and sauté the onions and garlic until soft and translucent. Add the minced meat and cook for 10–15 minutes until it is lightly browned. Add the rice, paprika, and parsley, stirring well for 2–3 minutes. Remove from the heat and set aside to cool to a manageable temperature.

3 Place a ball of the stuffing in the centre of a sauerkraut or cabbage leaf. Fold in the sides of the leaf and roll it up to form a closed parcel. Repeat with the rest of the stuffing and cabbage leaves.

4 Arrange a layer of sauerkraut in the bottom of a large saucepan with a lid, followed by the cabbage parcels, loose ends facing down, and topped with the smoked pork or bacon. Carefully add hot water to the pan until it half-covers the contents of the pan. If necessary, weigh the parcels down with a small heatproof plate. Put the lid on and simmer over a low heat for 2 hours or until cooked, making sure the water doesn't evaporate. The water should remain at the same level, half-covering the contents of the pan, throughout the cooking time.

5 Meanwhile, make the sauce. Heat the olive oil in a small saucepan, add the flour and allow to brown slightly, then add the salt, black peppercorns, tomato purée, chilli, crème fraîche, and enough water to make a sauce with the consistency of pouring cream. When the sauerkraut parcels are cooked, divide between 4 serving plates and pour some of the hot sauce over each portion.

Savoy Cabbage Parcels

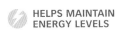 **HELPS MAINTAIN ENERGY LEVELS**　　 **HELPS BUILD MUSCLE**　　 **ENHANCES VIGOUR**　　 **CALMING AND COMFORTING**

This dish is great comfort food, but it is also packed with healthy ingredients that boost energy levels. It is a good choice for men of all ages, as quinoa provides protein and essential amino acids that help the body build muscle, while walnuts can help improve men's fertility and are heart-healthy. This also makes an ideal complete meal for vegetarians and vegans.

SERVES 4

300g (10oz) quinoa

60g (2oz) walnuts, roughly chopped

50g (1¾oz) sun-dried tomatoes, chopped

2 garlic cloves, finely chopped

1 medium red onion, finely chopped

4 small shallots, finely chopped

6 tbsp chopped parsley

100g (3½oz) fresh or dried unsweetened cranberries

2 tsp ground pimento

½ tsp ground coriander

2 level tsp Italian herbs seasoning

Himalayan salt and freshly ground black pepper

1 large Savoy cabbage, leaves removed

4 bay leaves

2 tsp plain flour, arrowroot, or kudzu (a popular Asian thickener)

thick natural yogurt, to serve

1 To make the stuffing, wash the quinoa grains, allow to drip-dry, and put in a mixing bowl with the walnuts, tomatoes, garlic, onion, shallots, parsley, and cranberries. Season with the pimento, ground coriander, Italian seasoning, and salt and black pepper, and combine all the ingredients thoroughly.

2 Choose 10–12 tender medium-sized cabbage leaves and blanch in boiling water for 1–2 minutes, removing them as soon as they wilt. Reserve the cabbage water. Allow the leaves to cool for a moment, then cut away the thick vein at the back of each leaf.

3 Place a spoonful of stuffing in the centre of a cabbage leaf. Fold in the sides of the leaf and roll it up to form a closed parcel. Repeat with the rest of the stuffing and cabbage leaves.

4 Tightly arrange the parcels, loose ends facing down, in the bottom of a medium saucepan with a lid. Layer the parcels if necessary, adding the bay leaves as you work.

5 Add the reserved cabbage water to the pan, making sure that the base of the pan is covered but the parcels are only partially covered with liquid. Bring to the boil, reduce the heat, put on the lid, and simmer gently for 30 minutes.

6 Dissolve the flour in a mug of water and add it to the pan. Simmer for another 15 minutes or until the sauce has thickened and the parcels are cooked. Serve accompanied with a spoonful of thick yogurt.

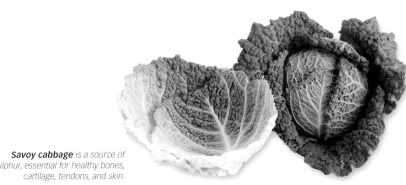

Savoy cabbage is a source of sulphur, essential for healthy bones, cartilage, tendons, and skin.

Wood Pigeon Breasts With Goji Berries

 HELPS MAINTAIN ENERGY LEVELS   **ENHANCES VIGOUR AND A SENSE OF WELL-BEING**   **REPLACES IRON LOST IN MENSTRUATION**   **HELPS TONE THE KIDNEYS**

Wood pigeon meat is lean, tender, and nutritious. In China, it is regarded as an excellent kidney tonic, but it is most commonly eaten to help combat male and female infertility by boosting blood circulation and improving energy levels. It also helps build iron levels after substantial blood loss, such as at childbirth or heavy menstruation. Goji berries are added to give a metabolic boost.

SERVES 4

4 whole pigeons

25g (scant 1oz) dried shiitake mushrooms

2 medium carrots, halved lengthways

1 medium onion, peeled and quartered

1 medium red chilli, whole

4 garlic cloves in their skins

½ tsp black peppercorns

a pinch of salt

4 tsp cornflour

20g (¾oz) goji berries

a dash of olive oil

coriander leaves, chopped, to garnish

1 Remove the breast meat in whole pieces from each bird and reserve. Place the filleted birds in a large casserole pot and add the mushrooms, carrots, onion, chilli, garlic, black peppercorns, and salt. Pour in enough water to just cover, bring it to the boil, and simmer over a low heat for 1½ hours, skimming off any impurities from the top of the stock as necessary. Watch the liquid level and add more water if needed. Towards the end of the cooking time, you should have approximately 500ml (16fl oz) or more of stock remaining.

2 Strain the stock, reserving the cooking liquid, shiitake mushrooms, garlic cloves, and some of the peppercorns. Discard the rest of the ingredients including the pigeon meat, bones, and skin. Shred the mushrooms and squeeze the softened garlic cloves from their skins. Set the garlic paste aside.

3 Return the stock to the casserole pot, reserving 4 tablespoons in a mug, and set over a medium-high heat. Thicken the liquid by mixing the cornflour with the reserved stock in the mug and adding it to the pot. Add the goji berries, shredded mushrooms, and the garlic paste and simmer the stock for 10–20 minutes until it thickens to the consistency of double cream. Adjust the seasoning if required.

4 Add a dash of olive oil to a frying pan and warm over a medium heat. Add the reserved pigeon breasts and pan-fry for 2 minutes on each side until just cooked through. Transfer to the casserole pot and cook for 2–3 minutes.

5 Arrange the breasts on a warm serving plate, spoon over a little of the sauce, and garnish with the coriander leaves. Serve with the remaining sauce in a jug and some boiled rice.

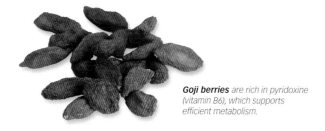

Goji berries are rich in pyridoxine (vitamin B6), which supports efficient metabolism.

Ginger Chicken

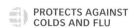 **PROTECTS AGAINST COLDS AND FLU**

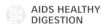 **AIDS HEALTHY DIGESTION**

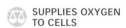 **SUPPLIES OXYGEN TO CELLS**

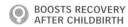 **BOOSTS RECOVERY AFTER CHILDBIRTH**

The marinade in this chicken dish contains fresh ginger, which is one of the most important foods for helping prevent and treat common colds. Its warming nature is enhanced here with lime, garlic, and honey – all known to help boost the immune system. This dish is ideal if you need to increase your resistance to seasonal bugs or build your strength after an illness.

SERVES 4

1 organic free-range chicken, approximately 1.5kg (3lb 3oz), cut into 8 pieces

1 tbsp ghee or clarified butter

1kg (2¼lb) potatoes, peeled and thinly sliced

½–1 tsp salt

1 tbsp paprika

½ tsp freshly ground black pepper

For the marinade

4 tbsp tamari soy sauce

1 heaped tbsp finely chopped fresh root ginger

3–5 garlic cloves, crushed

zest and juice of 1–2 limes

3 tbsp honey

1 Prepare the marinade by mixing the tamari soy sauce, ginger, garlic, lime juice, and honey in a clean plastic container with a lid. Add the chicken pieces and marinate for 8–12 hours or overnight in the refrigerator.

2 Preheat the oven to 220°C (425°F/Gas 7). Grease a large ovenproof dish with the ghee. Arrange the sliced potatoes in thin layers in the dish and sprinkle the salt, paprika, and black pepper on top. Place the chicken pieces on top of the potatoes. Pour any remaining marinade on top and season with salt and black pepper. Bake in the oven for 45–50 minutes or until the chicken juices run clear when the meat is pierced with a sharp knife, and the potatoes are cooked. Serve with salad.

Ghee is a good source of lauric acid, a healthy fat with antibacterial and antifungal properties.

Mushroom Frittata With Cherry Tomatoes And Basil

 HELPS STRENGTHEN THE IMMUNE SYSTEM   **AIDS HEALTHY DIGESTION**   **HELPS EASE RHEUMATIC PAIN**   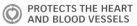 **PROTECTS THE HEART AND BLOOD VESSELS**

This is an ideal meal if you are convalescing. Like other mushrooms, morels (*Morchella esculenta*) are rich in the essential amino acids that the body needs to build protein, while shiitake and crimini mushrooms help improve digestion and have anti-inflammatory properties. Wash the morels thoroughly under running water, as their sponge-like caps often contain soil and grit.

SERVES 4

For the braised tomatoes

½ tbsp ghee, or clarified butter, for greasing

200g (7oz) ripe cherry tomatoes

salt and freshly ground black pepper

1 tbsp freshly chopped basil leaves, to garnish

For the frittata

25g (scant 1oz) dried morels, soaked in boiling water for 5 minutes to rehydrate, or 75g (2½oz) fresh morels, cleaned and finely chopped

100g (3½oz) shiitake mushrooms, sliced

100g (3½oz) crimini mushrooms, sliced

2 tbsp ghee

salt and freshly ground black pepper

2 tbsp finely chopped chives

8 eggs, beaten

3 tbsp crème fraîche

1 Preheat the oven to 180°C (350°F/Gas 4). To braise the tomatoes, grease a baking tray with the ghee, add the cherry tomatoes, season with salt and black pepper, and cook in the oven for 8–10 minutes or until the tomatoes are cooked.

2 Meanwhile, place a large, non-stick frying pan over a medium heat and dry-fry all the mushrooms for 1–2 minutes to enhance their flavour, and allow them to release some of their moisture. Add 1 tablespoon of the ghee, allow to melt, and sauté the mushrooms for 3–5 minutes, adding salt and black pepper to taste. Add half the chopped chives to the mushrooms, reserving the rest to use as a garnish. Remove the mushrooms from the pan and set aside.

3 Beat together the eggs and crème fraîche in a medium bowl with a little more salt and black pepper to taste. Melt the remaining tablespoon of ghee in the pan and pour in the egg mixture. Cook for 2–3 minutes over a low heat until the base is firm, then add the mushrooms and cover with a lid to cook for 3–5 minutes, until both the base and top of the frittata are set.

4 To serve, sprinkle the frittata with the rest of the chives, divide between 4 serving plates, and add the braised cherry tomatoes. Garnish the tomatoes with the basil and serve immediately.

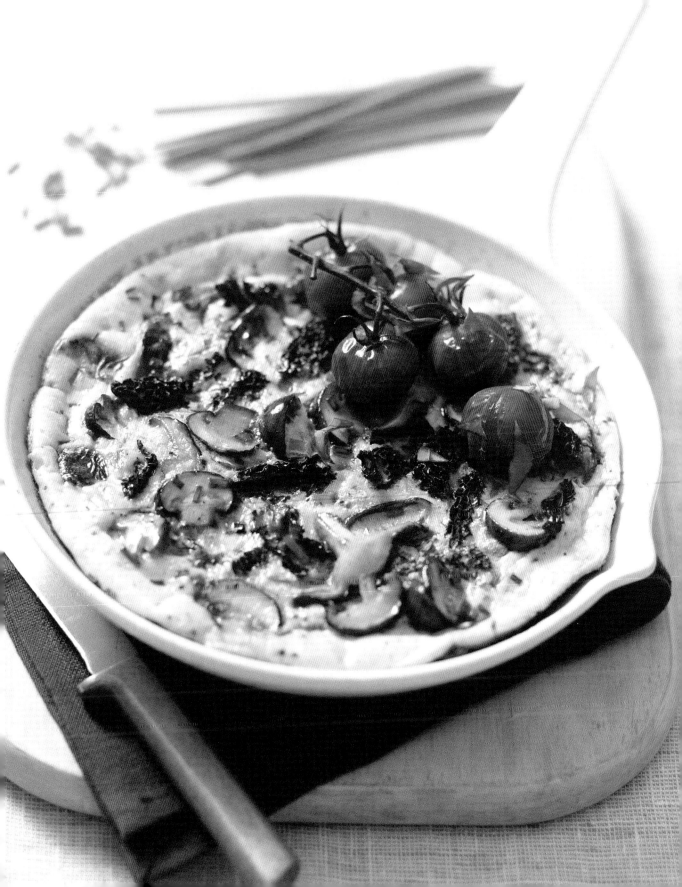

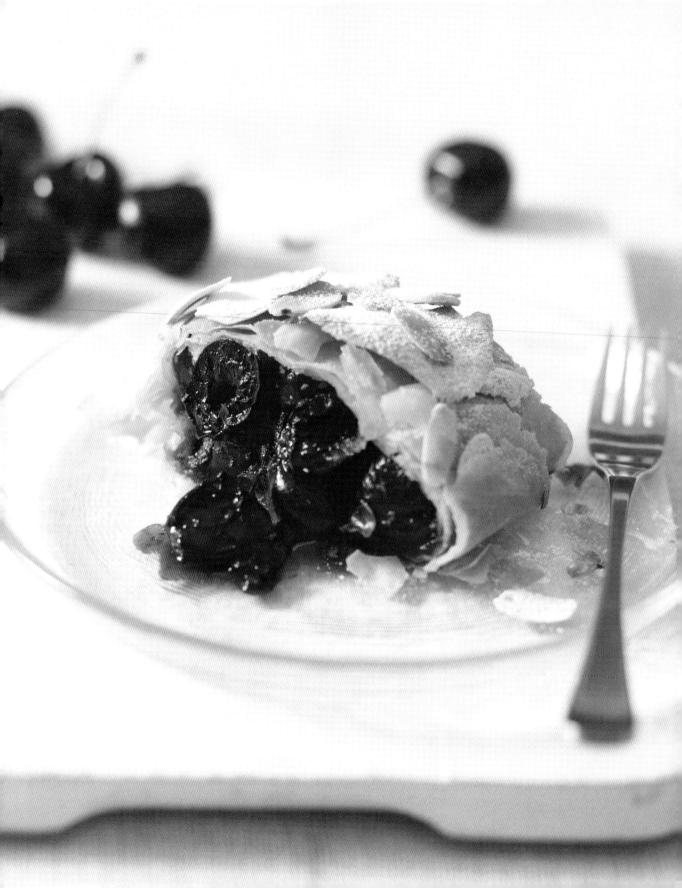

CHERRY STRUDEL

 PROTECTS AGAINST FREE-RADICAL DAMAGE

PROTECTS THE HEART AND BLOOD VESSELS

HELPS EASE JOINT INFLAMMATION

HELPS RELIEVE INSOMNIA

The tart morello cherries in this recipe are particularly rich in antioxidants which help protect the heart and fight free-radical damage and inflammation, especially in the joints. They also contain melatonin, which aids restful sleep. if you can't find morello cherries, choose a sweet variety and marinate in the zest of an orange and the juice of half a lemon for a sharper flavour.

SERVES 4

35g (1¼oz) fresh breadcrumbs

50g (1¾oz) caster sugar

25g (scant 1oz) ground almonds

25g (scant 1oz) ground walnuts

5 sheets ready-made filo pastry

35g (1¼oz) unsalted butter, melted, plus a little extra for brushing

½ tsp ground cinnamon

325g (11oz) fresh morello cherries, pitted

3 tbsp flaked almonds (optional)

icing sugar, for dusting

1 To make the filling, mix the breadcrumbs, caster sugar, and ground almonds together in a bowl and set aside.

2 Preheat the oven to 190°C (375°F/Gas 5). If you can't find ground walnuts, blitz some walnut pieces in a food processor or blender. Arrange a sheet of baking parchment on a flat surface. Lay a sheet of filo pastry on the parchment, with one of the longer edges of the pastry rectangle facing you. Brush the surface of the pastry with some of the melted butter and sprinkle over a little of the cinnamon. Repeat with the rest of the pastry sheets, butter, and cinnamon. Scatter the breadcrumb filling over the pastry stack, leaving a 5cm (2in) border around the edge (this will help when you fold the pastry edges over to prevent the filling escaping). If you want to make 2 strudels, cut the pastry in half, leaving a 10cm (4in) space in the middle. Scatter the ground walnuts over the filling and heap the cherries in a thick strip along the centre of the pastry, leaving a 5cm (2in) gap at either end.

3 Fold in the short edges of the pastry rectangle. Then, using the baking parchment, fold over the long edge of the pastry rectangle nearest you, and roll up the pastry to enclose the filling and create a long roll. Brush the surface of the rolled pastry with more melted butter and scatter over the flaked almonds, if using.

4 Lift the baking parchment with the strudel, seam-side down, onto a large baking sheet and bake in the oven for 30 minutes or until the pastry is golden. Allow to cool for about 10 minutes, then dust with icing sugar and serve.

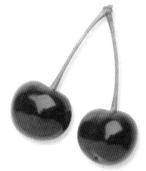

Morello cherries *are coloured brightly with red pigments that produce a greater pain-relieving effect than aspirin.*

ACKNOWLEDGMENTS

The authors would like to thank Peter Kindersley whose tireless support for organic food and a natural lifestyle helped to create this book. Thanks also to Daphne Lambert for recipe inspiration and feedback; to Alex Savage for assisting with research; and to all at Dorling Kindersley for helping to steer this volume from concept to completion.

Dorling Kindersley would like to thank the great team at Neal's Yard Remedies.

Recipe photography Stuart West
Art direction Kat Mead
Food styling Jane Lawrie
Prop styling Liz Hippisley
Additional ingredients photography Ian O'Leary
Proofreading Sue Morony, Kokila Manchanda, and Neha Ruth Samuel
Recipe testing Hülya Balci, Amy Carter, Francesa Dennis, Katy Greenwood, Clare Nielsen-Marsh, and Ann Reynolds
Editorial assistance Martha Burley
Design assistance Collette Sadler and Pooja Verma

All images © Dorling Kindersley
For further information see: **www.dkimages.com**

AUTHORS

Susan Curtis
Susan runs a busy practice as a homeopath and naturopath and is the Director of Natural Health for Neal's Yard Remedies. She is the author of several books, including Essential Oils, and co-author of Natural Healing for Women. Susan has two children and is passionate about helping people to live a more natural and healthy lifestyle.

Pat Thomas
Pat is a journalist, campaigner, and broadcaster. Her previous books include Cleaning Yourself to Death, What's in this Stuff?, and Skin Deep. Through her work she has led the way in exposing harmful chemicals in many everyday products, as well as promoting natural alternatives that work. She is a former editor of The Ecologist magazine and is a trustee of the Organic Research Centre and editor of Neal's Yard Remedies' natural health website, NYR Natural News.

Dragana Vilinac
A fourth-generation herbalist widely respected for her vast knowledge and expertise, Dragana's passion for herbal medicine has taken her around the world, and has led her to train in disciplines including Western Herbal Medicine and Traditional Chinese Medicine. Dragana is Head Herbalist for Neal's Yard Remedies.